NUTRITION
and HEALTH
Today

Second Edition

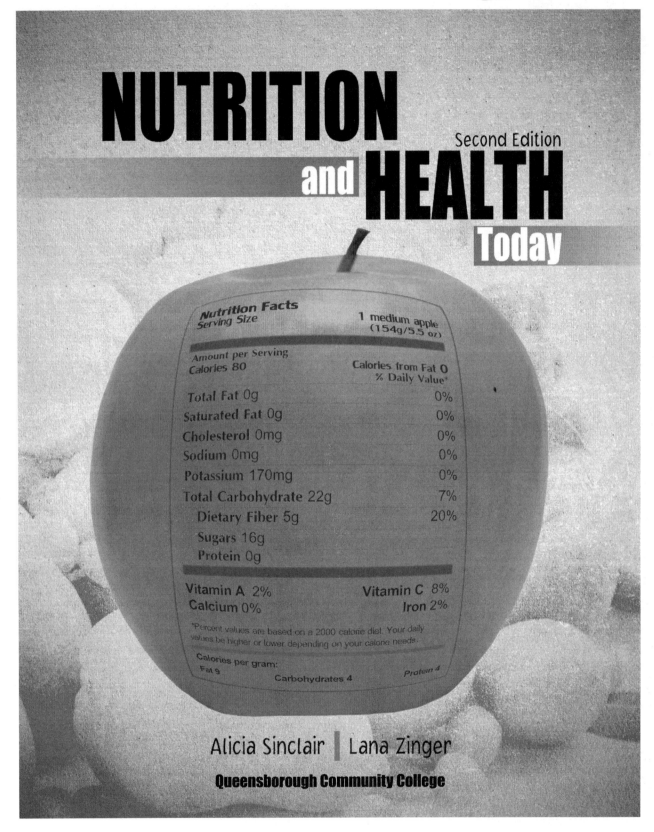

Nutrition Facts
Serving Size 1 medium apple
(154g/5.5 oz)

Amount per Serving
Calories 80   Calories from Fat 0
                                % Daily Value*

Total Fat 0g   0%
Saturated Fat 0g   0%
Cholesterol 0mg   0%
Sodium 0mg   0%
Potassium 170mg   0%
Total Carbohydrate 22g   7%
   Dietary Fiber 5g   20%
   Sugars 16g
   Protein 0g

Vitamin A 2%   Vitamin C 8%
Calcium 0%   Iron 2%

*Percent values are based on a 2000 calorie diet. Your daily
values be higher or lower depending on your calorie needs.

Calories per gram:
Fat 9
          Carbohydrates 4   Protein 4

Alicia Sinclair | Lana Zinger
Queensborough Community College

Kendall Hunt
publishing company

Previously titled: The Fundamentals of Nutrition & Health

Cover images © Shutterstock, Inc.

Kendall Hunt
publishing company

www.kendallhunt.com
Send all inquiries to:
4050 Westmark Drive
Dubuque, IA 52004-1840

Copyright © 2008, 2011 by Alicia Sinclair & Lana Zinger

ISBN 978-0-7575-9025-2

Printed in the United States of America
10 9 8 7 6 5 4 3 2

CONTENTS

1 Introduction to Nutrition   1

2 Dietary Guidelines for Americans   17

3 The Nutrients   35

4 Diet and Health   55

5 Lifecycle Nutrition   79

6 Diet and Nutrition Trends   95

7 Dangers in Our Food Supply   109

8 Obesity and Weight Management   131

9 Myths and Misconceptions   145

10 Eating Better in America: Putting It All Together!   159

11 Healthy Recipes   181

Index   209

chapter 1
Introduction to Nutrition

Nutrition is a much talked about subject. Every day, you hear nutrition messages from the media and sort through information from advertisers who want you to buy their products. Some products are healthy, but others may be lacking in nutrients. Sometimes it is difficult to sort it all out. Although many of us are aware that a healthy diet can prevent disease, not enough of us know about the healing powers of food. Proper nutrition helps regulate behavior, increase energy, and boost mood. With the right vitamins, minerals, essential fatty acids, and amino acids, people can begin to fight all sorts of conditions from cancer to heart disease. Nutrition awareness can help people make healthy food choices.

Maintaining Proper Nutrition Can:

- Give you stamina and energy for life
- Help you maintain an ideal body weight
- Boost your immune system
- Improve sports performance
- Delay the effects of aging
- Keep you active and fit into old age
- Help beat fatigue
- Protect teeth and keep gums healthy
- Enhance your ability to concentrate
- Alter mood
- Ward off serious illnesses like heart disease, certain cancers, diabetes type 2, and gallbladder disease

What Is Your Definition of Nutrition?

Brainstorm what you think about nutrition. What pops into your head? Do you have a negative or positive association? Where did you learn about nutrition?

_____

_____

_____

_____

_____

_____

_____

Ask someone what comes to mind when they hear the word *nutrition,* and most people respond: "diets," "vitamins," "healthy foods." Few people realize that nutrition is actually a science because nutrition as a discipline is fairly new. Nutrition has only been studied for roughly a century. People are bombarded with so many weight loss messages that few recognize it as a true science. In fact, **nutrition is a new science that borrows from other sciences (i.e., chemistry, anatomy and physiology, biochemistry, and microbiology) that looks at the relationship between the foods we eat and our health.**

To put a time frame into perspective, the 100 years since 1890 were a large period of growth of the science of nutrition. Several key events took place during 1907 to 1919:

- E. V. McCollum (Sommer, 1989) and Adelle Davis (Harper, 1991) discovered fat-soluble vitamin A in butter and discovered water-soluble vitamin B in wheat germ.
- Axel Holst and Theodor Frolich were pioneers in the combat of scurvy by discovering an antiscorbutic substance (vitamin C) in fresh vegetables (Norum & Gray, 2002).
- By experimenting with fish oils, Edward Mellanby discovered a substance (vitamin D) to prevent rickets (Mellanby & Cantag, 1919).

By 1920, the science of nutrition was beginning to add reliable information about relationships between diet and health. These pivotal "discoveries" set the stage for the next several decades of nutrient research.

Why Good Nutrition Is Important

- **People are dying from unhealthy eating and inactivity.** According to the U.S. Department of Health and Human Services, unhealthy eating and inactivity cause **310,000 to 580,000 deaths every year,** which is similar to the number of deaths caused by tobacco and 13 times more than are caused by guns.
- **Quality of life is reduced.** Unhealthy eating and physical inactivity are major contributors to reduced quality of life and disabilities.
- **Almost two-thirds (61%) of American adults are overweight or obese.** Obesity rates in children have doubled in the last two decades, prompting concern about the rates of diet- and inactivity-related diseases that will occur as obese children age.
- **Diet and inactivity-related diseases are expensive.** Better nutrition could reduce the cost of heart disease, cancer, stroke, and diabetes by **$71 billion** each year.

Good Nutrition Provides Energy

The foods that you eat provide the energy that your body needs to function. Just like you need to put fuel in your car or recharge your cell phone battery, your body needs to be fed energy-providing foods every day. The main form of energy for your body is carbohydrates.

Good Nutrition Provides Muscles

Protein in the foods you that eat is broken down into individual amino acids. Your body uses the amino acids to build and repair the various parts of your body. Your muscles contain lots of protein, and you must replenish that protein through your diet. Your body also needs protein for components of your immune system, hormones, nervous system, and organs.

Your body also needs fats to be healthy. Membranes that contain fats surround all the cells of your body. Your brain has fatty acids, and fats are also needed to signal hormones.

Good Nutrition Provides Vitamins, Minerals, and Other Helpers

Vitamins and minerals that you get from your diet are just as important as carbohydrates, protein, and fats; however, you only need vitamins and minerals in small amounts. Vitamins and minerals usually function as coenzymes, which mean they help chemical reactions in the body happen a lot faster. For example, many of the B complex vitamins help your body burn carbohydrates for energy. Vitamin A is needed for vision, zinc is involved in many metabolic processes, and vitamin C helps keep connective tissue strong and your immune system functioning.

Phytochemicals are found in the colorful parts of fruits and vegetables. Although they are not required for body functioning, they may have a very powerful impact on your health. For example, quercetin, which is found in red apples functions like an antihistamine and as an anti-inflammatory effect. Resveratrol, which is found in grape skins and seeds, is a powerful antioxidant. Antioxidants help protect your body from free radical damage that comes from the sun, pollution, smoke, and poor dietary choices. They are found in the phytochemicals of fruits and vegetables, as well as some vitamins and amino acids.

HOW POWERFUL IS A NUTRITIOUS DIET IN PREVENTING DISEASE?

So, is there a relationship between the foods that we eat and our health? You bet! Many disease states are associated with the foods that we eat. The choices that we make on a daily basis can, over time, wreak havoc on our health and have dire consequences. Malnutrition occurs if our bodies fail to get all the nutrients they need. If a person suffers from malnutrition he or she may be more likely to contract diseases. Malnutrition can affect the functions of their body such as brain, eyesight, organs, height, weight, as well as the formation of body parts if the child is still in its mother's womb. In the developing world, the biggest concerns often lie with the lack of vitamins and minerals, as well as the access to clean drinking water. According to the United Nations Children's Fund (UNICEF), almost one-third of children in developing countries are malnourished. In addition to the shortage of food, disease also causes malnutrition. Diseases such as diarrhea cause the body to lose essential nutrients, by flushing them out of the body. Nutrients can take a long time to replace and may affect a child's growth and development.

In the United States, malnutrition is less of a problem as over-nutrition and lifestyle diseases associated with eating too much or eating the wrong types of food. Lifestyle choices or modifiable behaviors are major causes of mortality in the United States. A lifestyle choice, or modifiable behavior is something that a person has some control over whether or not he or she will do that behavior.

In the United States, more than one-third of all deaths can be attributed to a limited number of largely preventable behaviors and exposures including smoking, poor diet, physical inactivity, and alcohol consumption. Like tobacco, obesity and inactivity increase the risks for the top three killers: heart disease, cancer, and cerebrovascular ailments including strokes. Obesity and inactivity also strongly increase the risk of diabetes, the sixth leading cause of death.

By the time they reach early adulthood, a large proportion of American youth have begun the poor practices contributing to three leading causes of preventable death in the United States: smoking, physical inactivity, and alcohol abuse. This finding is according to an analysis of the most comprehensive survey of adolescent health behavior undertaken to date by the National Institutes of Health (NIH). The analysis also found that significant health disparities exist between racial groups, and that Americans are less likely to have access to health care when they reach adulthood than they did during the teenage years.

Fast food and larger portions of it are taking a toll in the United States, where the surgeon general says 60 percent of adults are overweight or obese, as are nearly 13 percent of children. The prevalence of excess weight and obesity has nearly doubled among children and adolescents since 1980, and is increasing in both sexes and among all adults. The trends are already associated with major increases in the prevalence of conditions such as asthma and type 2 diabetes mellitus in children.

Changing modifiable behaviors can increase a person's life expectancy or longevity and prevent early deaths (McGinnis & Foege, 1993).

The following diseases are associated with poor diet:

- Hypertension
- Coronary artery disease
- Type II diabetes
- Osteoporosis
- Certain types of cancer, such as breast and colon cancer
- Obesity
- Elevated blood lipid levels

Number of deaths for leading causes of death

- Heart disease: 616,067
- Cancer: 562,875
- Stroke (cerebrovascular diseases): 135,952
- Chronic lower respiratory diseases: 127,924
- Accidents (unintentional injuries): 123,706
- Alzheimer's disease: 74,632
- Diabetes: 71,382
- Influenza and pneumonia: 52,717
- Nephritis, nephrotic syndrome, and nephrosis: 46,448
- Septicemia: 34,828

Source: *http://www.cdc.gov*

NUTRIENTS

The discipline of nutrition looks at the relationship between the foods we eat and one's health. Specifically, nutrition is concerned with *nutrients*.

Nutrients are substances found in food that help promote the growth and maintenance of the body.

When thinking about "growth and maintenance" of the body, many people think, "But, I'm *done* growing!" And, for people 18 years and older, this is true in its literal sense. However, the human body is growing and maintaining on a daily basis. The foods that we eat, which are made up of nutrients, help the body perform vital functions on a cellular level. For example, hair, skin, and nails are all made up of the nutrients in the foods we eat. Nutrients (such as protein) also help make certain hormones, like insulin, which helps regulate our blood sugar levels. We literally become the nutrients that we eat! If you eat a lot of junk food, your body's tissues are unhealthy. If you eat a lot of good-for-you foods, your body's tissues are healthy.

Six essential nutrients exist. "Essential" here means that the body cannot make nutrients on its own. In other words, the only way for us to get nutrients is by eating them. Each nutrient will be discussed in more detail in later chapters.

1. **Carbohydrate**
   Carbohydrates are the body's preferred fuel source and are found in plant-based foods like pasta, bread, rice, and fruits and vegetables.

2. **Lipid**
   Lipid is the chemical name for a family of fatty substances. In other words, lipids are fats and oils. Examples include different plant oils like olive or canola. Butter and lard are also examples of a lipid.

3. **Protein**
   Protein helps build and repair the body. Foods rich in protein include beef, poultry, fish, dairy, eggs, and some plant foods like beans and nuts.

4. **Vitamins**
   Vitamins are substances the body needs in small amounts. Vitamins, along with minerals, act like spark plugs on a car's engine. Vitamins help the body perform vital tasks and prevent serious illness. Examples include vitamins A, D, E, K, and C; folate; niacin; thiamin; and riboflavin.

5. **Minerals**
   Minerals are substances the body needs in small amounts. Some examples include calcium, fluoride, and iodine.

6. **Water**
   Water is absolutely vital to all bodily functions. Water can be consumed in its pure form or through other beverages like milk, juice, or tea.

The first three nutrients—*carbohydrate*, *lipids*, and *protein*—are a little different than the last three (vitamins, minerals, and water). They are often collectively referred to as "energy-yielding nutrients." Think of energy not as in "Rah, Rah! I'm so excited and energetic!" but instead think of **energy** as:

The capacity to do work.

What kind of "work" do you do each day? Take a moment and list all the activities that you do (for example, I walk to class). All of this work requires energy that allows you to move from point A to point B. This all happens because of the energy-yielding nutrients. Carbohydrates, lipid, and protein are considered energy yielding specifically because they contain calories and break them down to yield energy the body can use. For our purposes, you can think of a **calorie** as:

The measurement of a food's energy value.

On a more scientific level, a calorie is a measurement of heat. Specifically, food energy is measured in kilocalories (1,000 calories equal 1 kilocalorie) often abbreviated kcalories or kcal. A capitalized version is also sometimes used: Calories. One **kcalorie** is

The amount of heat necessary to raise the temperature of 1 kilogram (kg) of water 1 degree Celsius (Whitney & Rolfes, 1996).

The energy content of a particular food depends on how much of each of the energy-yielding nutrients it contains. Once completely broken down in the body, 1 gram (g) of carbohydrate yields about 4 kilocalories of energy; a gram of protein also yields 4 kcalories and 1 gram of lipid yields 9 calories! This is *more than* twice as many calories as a gram of carbohydrate or protein, respectively!

One other substance yields energy once when broken down in the body, yet it is not considered a nutrient because it does not help promote the growth and maintenance of the body (remember the definition of nutrient previously discussed): alcohol. One gram of alcohol yields 7 kilocalories. Quite a lot!

Remember the following list:

1 gram of carbohydrate = 4 kilocalories
1 gram of protein = 4 kilocalories
1 gram of lipid = 9 kilocalories
1 gram of alcohol = 7 kilocalories

Let's say you have a Mystery Candy Bar. It contains 22 grams of carbohydrate, 3 grams of protein, and 12 grams of lipid. How many total kilocalories does it contain?

$22g \times 4 = 88$
$3g \times 4 = 12$
$12g \times 9 = 108$
TOTAL = 208 kcals

Let's try another one:

A Mystery Bag of Chips contains 31 grams of carbohydrate, 4 grams of protein and 10 grams of lipid. How many total kilocalories does it contain?

$31g \times ??$
$4g \times ??$
$10g \times ??$
TOTAL = ??

Many people have the misconception that vitamins and minerals are what give them energy. Have you ever felt tired or run down and been told, "Oh, you just need your vitamins." Nothing could be further from the truth. Vitamins and minerals do not yield energy in the body once broken down. Because of this, they cannot provide you with the capacity to do work. So we've just "busted" a myth: **vitamins and minerals do not provide or enhance energy!**

Another key point when learning about the six essential nutrients is to recognize that protein and carbohydrate contain the same kilocalories per gram. This is surprising to people especially given the anti-carbohydrate craze currently popular in the United States. Keep in mind that one gram of lipid contains more than twice as many kilocalories as a gram each of carbohydrate and protein.

What does this mean for weight loss and/or weight gain? More will be discussed in later chapters, but for now, remember the following:

If you consume more food calories than your body requires, those calories will be stored as fat; if you consume fewer calories than your body requires, your body will draw on stored fat reserves and you will lose weight.

Does this mean a person can gain weight by eating apples? Yes! Although it is much harder to gain weight eating apples than, say, a candy bar, if you consume more food calories than your body needs, no matter where it comes from, you store it as body fat.

How Many Calories Do You Need?

Each person has an allotted caloric value. In other words, each of us needs a certain amount of food in a given 24-hour time period. This amount is *highly variable* from person to person. Still, there are three main factors that help determine the number of food calories that should be eaten every day. Those factors are:

1. **Thermic Effect of Food:** this is the energy expended by the body simply to digest and absorb food. You burn roughly 5 to 10 percent due to the thermic effect of food. In other words, if you need 2,000 calories to maintain your current weight, you can assume that roughly 100 to 200 of those calories will be expended, thanks to the thermic effect of food.

2. **Physical Activity:** has a significant impact on energy expenditure and contributes roughly 20 to 30 percent to the body's total energy output. In other words, the more physically active you are, the more food calories you require to maintain your current weight.

    Think about it: who burns more calories each day? Someone who has a desk job or someone whose job requires a lot of footwork like a nurse or a construction worker? Simply put, the more physically active you are, the more food you are able to consume and still maintain your weight.

3. **Basal Metabolic Rate**
    Most of the body's energy, about 60 to 70 percent, goes to supporting the ongoing metabolic work of the body's cells. This includes such activities as heart beat, respiration, and maintaining body temperature. Basal metabolic rate is the amount of calories that your body requires in a state of rest. Let's say you are in a car accident tomorrow and you are in the hospital lying in a coma. Do you still need to eat? Of course!

What do you need the calories for if you are just lying there? All of your body's involuntary activities, like your kidneys filtering, heart pumping, and intestines digesting, require "fuel" to take place.

Several factors affect your body's basal metabolic rate, and these factors are what make each of us different.

-   **Height**
    In general, the taller a person is, the higher their basal metabolic rate. Imagine if you owned a small studio apartment and a four-floor townhouse. Which property would require more fuel to heat? The townhouse would because taller structures simply have more surface area and, as a result, require a lot of fuel.

-   **Body Temperature**
    Have you ever heard the old wives' tale, "Feed a fever, starve a cold"? A person with a fever has a slightly increased basal metabolic rate. Normal body temperature is 98.6 degrees Fahrenheit. For every one degree above normal body temperature, basal metabolic rate increases roughly 7 percent.

-   **Pregnancy and Lactation**
    Basal metabolic rate rises during pregnancy. In fact, after the first trimester of pregnancy, a woman requires an additional 300 kilocalories per day. Similarly, breastfeeding burns roughly an additional 500 kilocalories per day.

- **Growth**

  If you build a new skyscraper, what are some of the raw materials you would need to do so? Nails, cement, metal, screws, plaster board, etc. If you "build" a child, what are some of the raw materials necessary? FOOD! When a child is essentially growing from a "single story house" to a "skyscraper," the basal metabolic rate will rise to accommodate this.

- **Physical Activity**

  Through physical activity, especially strength training, basal metabolic rate rises. This factor is especially important because it is the one over which we truly have control.

Below is a simple formula to determine your daily calorie needs that takes into account all three of the above components.

For sedentary people: Weight × 14 = estimated calories/day

For moderately active people (exercise 3 days/week): Weight × 15 = estimated calories/day

For active people (exercise 5 days/week): Weight × 16 = estimated calories/day

---

To lose weight, you must create a caloric deficit preferably through both diet and exercise. It is recommended that you aim to lose one to two pounds per week. ***One pound of body fat contains 3,500 calories.*** So, if you wanted to lose one pound of body fat in one week, you would need to subtract 250 food calories from the above number you got and burn 250 calories most days of the week through physical activity. This would roughly create a 500 calorie per day deficit. 500 × 7 days in a week = 3,500.

Example:

Jane is 5′6″ and weighs 172 pounds. She is busy but not active and, therefore, realizes that she is sedentary.

$$172 \times 14 = 2,408$$

Jane is consuming roughly 2,400 calories to maintain her current weight of 172 pounds. In order to lose weight, she will need to cut her food intake by 250 calories per day and burn extra calories through exercise. A 45-minute power walk would burn roughly 250 calories.

So, instead of eating her normal 2,400 calories, Jane will eat roughly 2,150 (2,400 − 250 = 2,150). Instead of being sedentary, Jane will work out 4 to 5 days per week or more, increasing her energy expenditure. This will result in a one pound weight loss per week.

WHY DO WE EAT THE FOODS WE DO?

Every day, people make food choices, often without giving it much thought. Do you ever think about why you eat? The easy answers are because you are hungry, tired, and your stomach is rumbling. Sometimes you might eat because you are bored, sad, or happy; because it's lunchtime; or because that donut looks so good. Yet, if you dig a little deeper, most people have reasons behind their food selections whether they realize them or not.

Taste

Many people choose foods on taste alone. If it tastes good, eat it! Taste is largely determined by our genetics (Drayna, 2005). In other words, you've inherited a taste predisposition from your parents.

Children under 6 years old have abundant amounts of highly sensitive taste buds, which helps explain why they're often picky eaters. It is crucial that parents keep offering children, especially toddlers, a new food over and over again. Experts in pediatric nutrition point out that it may take up to 15 to 20 times for some children to be exposed to a food before they decide they like it.

When it comes to introducing new foods, the example set by you and by your child's peers can play a significant role. What kids see you eat becomes more acceptable to them. They are also more open to things they see other kids eating.

Cost

After taste, cost is a major factor behind food selection. The year 2008 has seen significant shifts in food costs. Sky-high food prices are being seen globally. In Pakistan, wheat is being stockpiled and its military is guarding flour mills. Indonesian consumers have taken to the streets to protest rising soy prices. Malaysia no longer lets people take sugar, flour, or cooking oil out of the country. North Dakota, the top U.S. wheat-producing state, may import from Canada due to tight supplies (Kirchoff & Waggoner, 2008).

Soaring demand along with rising oil prices have sent many commodity prices to their highest levels in history. Prices for some varieties of wheat are at an all-time high of more than $16 a bushel on the Minneapolis Grain Exchange. Corn, which has averaged about $2.50 per bushel in recent years, is above $5 in 2008.

According to the Bureau of Labor Statistics, in 2006, bread cost $1.05 per pound. In 2008, bread cost $1.28 per pound. Apples in 2006 cost 96 cents per pound. In 2008, they cost $1.16 per pound. In 2006, a dozen eggs cost $1.45. In 2008, they cost $2.18.

What does all of this mean for consumers? Unfortunately, as Americans face these rising food costs, more and more people will turn to unhealthy, low-quality sources, like fast-food restaurants and vending machines (Frazao, 1999). They may also skip meals altogether or forgo staples such as bread and dairy.

One way to combat soaring food costs is to shop at local green markets, a trend that has increased in the past decade. Green markets offer fresh, locally grown foods that tend to be cheaper than regular grocery stores because the food didn't have to be shipped long distances.

Convenience and Availability

In addition to financial feasibility, people eat foods that are accessible, quick, and easy to prepare. In 2006, Americans reported eating out approximately five times a week. Fast-food restaurants were the most popular eating establishments for breakfast and lunch, and fast-food and casual dining were the two most popular places for dinner. Ease, convenience, and cost were among the top reasons respondents ordered value/combo meals at fast-food restaurants (*Science Daily*, 2007). Unfortunately, all of this eating out can lead to dire health consequences.

Emotional Comfort

Americans are notorious for their love of food. We eat when we are happy, sad, angry, bored, lonely, anxious, and depressed. The one time we *should* eat is when we are truly hungry and we often don't. Hunger is the biological urge to eat, which is often felt below the neck. Appetite, on the other hand, is the psychological urge to eat, often "felt" above the neck. When people regularly consume food for comfort, it can lead to obesity and all of the health problems associated with overweight and obesity.

Culture/Family Background

Among the strongest factors behind food selection is a person's ethnic and cultural heritage. Simply put, people eat the foods they grew up eating.

Health and Body Weight

With more than 60 percent of adult Americans overweight or obese, it is no surprise that body weight is a factor behind a person's food selection. It's vital, however, that the person has a firm grasp on basic nutritional principles to help make healthy food choices.

What Does a Nutritious Diet Look Like?

Americans are always looking for a "quick fix" or the latest diet to follow or pill to take to solve their weight woes. In fact, a nutritious diet in its most simple form is easy to follow and has four basic characteristics. They are:

1. **Adequate**
   Adequate is a word that does not often come to mind, but in fact, most Americans are malnourished. They eat a lot, but a lot of the *wrong* foods. An adequate diet is one that ensures enough of the "good stuff" like fiber, protein, fruits, vegetables, and whole grains. An adequate diet limits, or avoids altogether, foods that are highly processed or refined.

2. **Balanced**
   Think back to when you learned about the different food groups. A balanced diet is one that incorporates all five food groups:
   • Fruits
   • Vegetables, including legumes and nuts
   • Whole grains
   • Low-fat dairy
   • Lean meats, poultry, and seafood
     Diets that propose eliminating an entire food group are not balanced and, unless there is a medical reason for doing so, can result in poor health.

3. **Varied**
   The term varied is sometimes confused with balanced, but they are different concepts as they relate to a person's diet. A varied diet includes a wide selection of foods. For example, say you bring a red delicious apple with you to lunch every day. One way to vary this would be to bring a golden delicious apple one day, and the next day bring a granny smith apple, and the next day try switching to a new fruit altogether! Do not be afraid to experiment with eating new foods. The point is that by eating a varied diet, you ensure that you are consuming many different nutrients.

4. **Moderate**
   Moderate is probably the most important characteristic of all. Look at the diets of other countries. The French, for example, eat a wide selection of foods such as fruits, vegetables, and whole grains, but they also consume butter, chocolate, and cheese. Then why are they

so slim compared to Americans? Moderation is the answer. A moderate diet is one that avoids excess. In other words, you may include your favorite "junk" foods in your daily diet. In fact, doing so means you are less likely to binge on these foods. The key, however, is to do so in moderation. Have one or two cookies, not the whole sleeve. Have a scoop of ice cream, not the whole pint. Have a slice or two of pizza, not the whole pie. One way to practice this is by listening to your body's cues. It will tell you when it is hungry. It will also tell you when it is satisfied. Once you get used to this—and it may take some time, especially if you are a member of the "clean your plate club"—your weight will naturally fall within its normal range.

This is really all healthy eating boils down to—an adequate, balanced, varied, and moderate diet. If you were to follow these principles, along with some moderate exercise, your weight should fall in a normal range for your height and genetics. The next time you, a friend, or a family member want to jump on the latest diet craze, remember these four characteristics, which will sustain you for life.

Because we are bombarded with nutrition news in newspapers, magazines, television, online, or just by talking with friends, it's more important than ever that we can believe in and safely use nutrition news we hear about. Unfortunately, the "expert" most people turn to for nutrition advice (i.e., a doctor) may not be the best person to help guide you. Only about one-fourth of all medical schools in the United States require students to take even one nutrition course (Shils, 1994). Today this is changing slowly, but surely. Still, physicians are burdened with many responsibilities and few will take the time, or truly have the expertise, to develop detailed diet plans for their patients. Instead, physicians often refer patients to registered dieticians, who are the appropriate qualified nutrition experts.

What Is a Registered Dietitian?

A registered dietician has the educational background necessary to deliver nutrition education and advice. To become a registered dietitian, a person must follow a rigorous bachelor's degree program with an emphasis in the sciences and clinical nutrition courses. During the final year of the bachelor's training, the student will follow a two-semester internship at various sites: clinical, community, and food service. Once these requirements have been met, the student must pass a national certification exam, indicating competency in core areas of dietetics.

By educating people about the connection between food and health, nutritionists and dietitians promote good eating habits to help prevent disease and to treat preexisting conditions.

Responsibilities of a Clinical Dietician

(Adapted by Whitney & Rolfes, 1996)

- Assesses clients' nutrition status.
- Determines clients' nutrient requirements.
- Monitors clients' nutrient intakes.
- Develops, implements, and evaluates clients' nutrition care plans.
- Counsels clients to cope with unique diet plans.
- Teachers clients and their families about nutrition and diet plans.
- Provides training for other dietitians, nurses, interns, and dietetics students.
- Serves as a liaison between clients and the food service department.
- Communicates with physicians, nurses, pharmacists, and other health care professionals about clients' progress, needs, and treatments.
- Participates in professional activities to enhance knowledge and skill.

Careers in Dietetics

Registered Dietitians work in a variety of settings including hospitals and other health care organizations, outpatient clinics, private practice, communication and public relations firms, government agencies including the military, and in education and school systems.

RESOURCES

Bureau of Labor Statistics: *http://www.bls.gov/* p. 13, 3rd paragraph.

Drayna, D. 2005. *Human Taste Genetics.* (6):217–235.

Frazao, E. High Costs of Poor Eating Patterns in the United States. In *America's Eating Habits: Changes and Consequences.* Economic Research Service, U.S. Department of Agriculture. Washington, DC: USDA, 1999. Agriculture Information Bulletin No. 750, 5–32.

Harper, A. E. 1991. *American Journal of Clinical Nutrition* 53:413–20.

Kirchhoff, S., Waggoner, J. 2008. *USA Today,* February 11.

McGinnis, J. M., Foege, W. H. 1993. Actual Causes of Death in the United States. *Journal of the American Medical Association.* 270 (18):2207–2212.

Mellanby, E. & Cantag, M. D. 1919. Experimental investigation on rickets. *Lancet* 196:407–412.

Norum, K. R., Gray, H. J. 2002. Axel Holst and Theodor Frolich—Pioneers in the combat of scurvy. *Tidsskr Nor Laegeforen* (June 30) 122 (17):1686–7.

Science Daily: Price and taste trump nutrition when Americans eat out. October 23, 2007.

Shils, M. E. 1994. Nutrition education in medical schools—the prospect before us. *American Journal of Clinical Nutrition* (Oct) 60 (4):631–8.

Sommer, A. 1989. New Imperatives for an Old Vitamin. *Journal of Nutrition* 119 (1):96–100.

United Nations Children's Fund (UNICEF). *http://www.unicef.org/index.php*

United States National Center for Health Statistics. 2007. *Health, United States.*

Whitney, E. N., Rolfes, S. R. 1996. *Understanding Nutrition* 7th ed. West Publishing Company.

chapter 2
Dietary Guidelines for Americans

HISTORY OF USDA'S FOOD GUIDANCE

The U.S. Department of Agriculture (USDA) has had a long history with food guidance dating back into the early twentieth century. Looking back over this history, many different food guides have been used. All of these food guides preceded the introduction of the original food guide pyramid in 1992.

1916: Food for Young Children
1940s: National Food Guide (commonly called "The Basic Seven")
1950s–1960s: Food for Fitness—A Daily Food Guide (commonly called "The Basic Four")
1970s: Hassle-Free Guide to a Better Diet
1992: Food Guide Pyramid
2005: MyPyramid

Before vitamins and minerals were even discovered, the USDA published its first dietary recommendations to the nation in 1894. In 1916, the first food guide, called Food for Young Children was published. Caroline Hunt, a nutritionist and the author, divided food into five groups: milk/meat, cereals, vegetables/fruits, fats/fatty foods, and sugars/sugary foods. Prompted by President Franklin Roosevelt, a National Nutrition Conference was called to action in 1941. For the first time, the USDA came up with Recommended Dietary Allowances (RDA's) for Americans to follow. In 1943, the USDA announced the "Basic Seven," which was a special modification of the nutritional guidelines to help people deal with the shortage of food supplies during the war.

Because of the complexity of the Basic Seven, the Basic Four was introduced and was used for the next 20 years. Milk, meats, fruits and vegetables, and grain products were the categories from which to eat foods. With chronic diseases like stroke and heart disease on the rise, the USDA needed to address the roles of unhealthy foods. During the late 1970s, the USDA added a fifth category to the Basic Four: fats, sweets, and alcoholic beverages, for people to consume in moderation.

Although a "Pattern for Daily Food Choices," the USDA's food guide, had been published annually since the 1980s, many people were still not aware that it existed. Beginning in 1988, the USDA created a graphic to represent the food groups. The USDA needed to convey the three main ideas: variety, proportionality, and moderation. The Food Guide Pyramid was finally released in 1992. Both the graphics and text conveyed variety and proportionality with pictures of foods and the size of the food group. In 1994, the Nutrition Labeling and Education Act required that every food in the grocery store have a nutritional label.

The Food Guide Pyramid

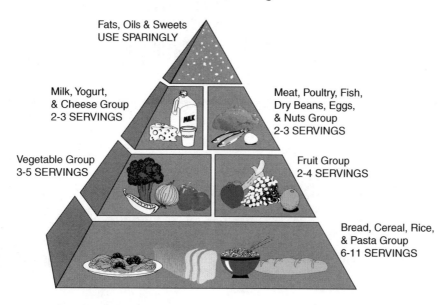

Source: http://wwwe.nal.usda.gov/fnic/Fpyr/pmap.htm

The Food Guide Pyramid was published in 1992 to replace the earlier food groups' classification system. Since that time, there has been an epidemic increase in type 2 diabetes which is now even afflicting a large and rapidly increasing number of children. The Food Guide Pyramid is an outline of what to eat each day based on the Dietary Guidelines. It is not a rigid prescription but instead a general guide that lets you choose a healthful diet that's right for you. The Pyramid calls for eating a variety of foods to get the nutrients you need and, at the same time, the right amount of calories to maintain healthy weight.

FAULTS OF THE USDA'S PYRAMID

Since the pyramid was released by the U.S. Department of Agriculture in 1992, nutrition scientists have criticized the content and design and proposed numerous alternatives, including the Harvard's Healthy Eating Pyramid. According to many scientists, the food pyramid is not up-to-date with current nutritional research. Harvard scientist Dr. Willet believes six faults of the food pyramid are misleading American people. Source: Willet, W. (2005) *Eat, Drink and Be Healthy: The Harvard Medical School Guide to Healthy Eating.*

1. **All fats are bad.** Not true! Only certain fats are bad for you (saturated and trans fats), while others (monosaturated and polyunsaturated fats) provide many benefits to your heart. Some of these good fats are found in nuts, fish, olive oil, and whole grains.

2. **All complex carbohydrates are good.** Not true! The food pyramid recommends six to eleven servings of carbohydrates a day, which is way too much. It also does not differentiate between the two kinds of carbohydrates, simple carbohydrates (sugars) and complex carbohydrates (starches). The majority of a person's carbohydrate intake should come from whole grains (complex carbs), which will make you feel fuller longer and also give you a lot of fiber. Stay away from refined carbohydrates, which are things like cookies, crackers, and chips. If you eat those, eat them in moderation.

3. **Protein is protein.** Not true! Protein should be a key component of your diet. But some sources of protein are better for you than others. For example, red meat (steaks) may have a good amount of protein, but they also are high in cholesterol and saturated fat, which is not good for your heart. Fish, chicken, turkey, and pork are lower in saturated fat and have just as much protein. Even beans and nuts are great sources of protein that people wouldn't necessarily know about.

4. **Dairy products are essential.** Not true! Dr. Willett says that despite all the commercials advertising protection against osteoporosis, there really is not a calcium emergency in America. Our country gets more calcium than any other country. In reality, he says, there are even studies that suggest that drinking and/or eating a lot of dairy sources can possibly increase a man's chance of getting prostate cancer or a woman's chance of getting ovarian cancer. You still need some calcium in your diet, however you don't have to get it from milk or yogurt. Spinach, tofu, orange juice, and broccoli have calcium and extra nutrients. A calcium supplement, which may be cheaper and lower in calories than dairy products, is another way to add calcium to a diet.

5. **Eat your potatoes.** Not true! Potatoes are starches, not vegetables! A baked potato increases blood sugar levels and insulin faster and to higher levels than an equal amount of calories from pure table sugar. French fries are even worse. If you must eat potatoes, eat them in moderation.

6. **No guidance on weight, exercise, alcohol, and vitamins.** Although the food pyramid suggests how to plan a healthy diet, it does not mention four other key parts of maintaining a healthy body: the importance of not gaining weight, the necessity of daily exercise, the potential health benefits of a daily alcoholic drink, and what you can gain by taking a daily multivitamin.

The Harvard School of Public Health created an alternative to the USDA's food pyramid called the Healthy Eating Pyramid. One of the most interesting changes in this pyramid is that plant oils are half of the near bottom part of the pyramid shared with grains. Harvard is stressing the importance of the right fats and the fact that fat calories make up about 30 percent of a healthy diet. The inclusion on exercise and maintaining a healthy weight are very important aspects of nutrition and are stressed in the Healthy Eating Pyramid by putting these as the base.

Tips for Using the Harvard's Healthy Eating Pyramid

1. **Start with exercise.** A healthy diet is built on a base of regular exercise, which keeps calories in balance and weight in check.

2. **Focus on food, not grams.** The Healthy Eating Pyramid does not address specific servings or grams of food, so neither should you. It is a simple, general guide to how you should eat when you eat.

3. **Go with plants.** Eating a plant-based diet is healthiest. Choose plenty of vegetables, fruits, whole grains, and healthy fats, like olive and canola oil.

4. **Cut way back on American staples.** Red meat, refined grains, potatoes, sugary drinks, and salty snacks are part of American culture, but they are also really unhealthy. Go for a plant-based diet rich in non-starchy vegetables, fruits, and whole grains. If you eat meat, fish and poultry are the best choices.

5. **Take a multivitamin, and maybe have a drink.** Taking a multivitamin can be a good nutrition insurance policy. Moderate drinking for many people can have real health benefits, but it is not for everyone. Moderate alcohol consumption is defined as two drinks or less per day for men and one drink or less per day for women. One drink equals one shot, one beer or 4 oz of wine. Those who don't drink shouldn't feel that they need to start.

BASIC PRINCIPLES OF ALL FOOD PYRAMIDS

With the variety of food pyramids available, you may wonder which one to follow. It may help to know that the basic principles of food pyramids are largely the same and generally emphasize the following:

- Eat more fruits, vegetables, and whole grains.
- Reduce intake of saturated fat, trans fat, and cholesterol.
- Limit sweets and salt.
- Drink alcoholic beverages in moderation, if at all.
- Control portion sizes and the total number of calories that you consume.
- Include physical activity in your daily routine.
- Food pyramids place foods in categories such as dairy products or meat and beans, to help guide your food choices. No single food provides all of the nutrients that your body needs, so eating a variety of foods within each group ensures that you get the necessary nutrients and other substances that promote good health.

THE DIETARY GUIDELINES FOR AMERICANS

The *Dietary Guidelines for Americans* has been published jointly every five years since 1980 by the Department of Health and Human Services (HHS) and the Department of Agriculture (USDA). The *Dietary Guidelines for Americans* provide research-based dietary advice designed to promote health and reduce risk for the major chronic conditions and diseases that affect people in the United States, including obesity, diabetes, cardiovascular disease, high blood pressure, cancer, and osteoporosis. The Dietary Guidelines are the cornerstone of federal nutrition policy and influence the numerous food and nutrition programs of the federal government. These include the Food Stamp Program; Special Supplemental Nutrition Program for Women, Infants, and Children (WIC); National School Lunch Program; and School Breakfast Program. The latest edition of the dietary guidelines was introduced in 2005.

Two-thirds of Americans are overweight or obese, and more than 50 percent of Americans do not get the recommended amount of physical activity. In 2005 guidelines emphasize physical activity and calorie control more than ever before.

The dietary guidelines describe a healthy diet as one that:

- Emphasizes fruits, vegetables, whole grains, and fat-free or low-fat milk and milk products;
- Includes lean meats, poultry, fish, beans, eggs, and nuts; and
- Is low in saturated fats, trans fats, cholesterol, salt (sodium), and added sugars.

MyPyramid replaces the Food Guide Pyramid introduced in 1992. MyPyramid is part of an overall food guidance system that emphasizes the need for a more individualized approach to improving diet and lifestyle. The new food guidance system utilizes interactive technology found on *www.mypyramid.gov.* The interactive activities make it easy for individuals to enter their age, gender, and physical activity level to obtain a more personalized recommendation on their daily calorie level based on the 2005 *Dietary Guidelines for Americans.* The web site features MyPyramid Plan, MyPyramid Tracker, and Inside MyPyramid, as well as tips, resources, as well as a worksheet.

MyPyramid.gov

MyPyramid food plans are designed for the general public ages 2 and over; they are not therapeutic diets.

ANATOMY OF MYPYRAMID

One Size Does Not Fit All

MyPyramid offers personalized eating plans, interactive tools to help you plan and assess your food choices, and advice to help you:

- Make smart choices from every food group.
- Find your balance between food and physical activity.
- Get the most nutrition out of your calories.
- Stay within your daily calorie needs.

Activity

Activity is represented by the steps and the person climbing them, as a reminder of the importance of daily physical activity.

Moderation

Moderation is represented by the narrowing of each food group from bottom to top. The wider base stands for foods with little or no solid fats or added sugars. These should be selected more often. The narrower top area stands for foods containing more added sugars and solid fats. The more active you are, the more of these foods can fit into your diet.

Personalization

Personalization is shown by the person on the steps, the slogan, and the URL, or web address. Find the kinds of and amounts of food to eat each day at MyPyramid.gov.

Proportionality

Proportionality is shown by the different widths of the food group bands. The widths suggest how much food a person should choose from each group. The widths are just a general guide, not exact proportions. Check the web site for how much is right for you.

Variety

Variety is symbolized by the six color bands representing the five food groups of the Pyramid and oils. This illustrates that foods from all groups are needed each day for good health.

Gradual Improvement

Gradual improvement is encouraged by the slogan. It suggests that individuals can benefit from taking small steps to improve their diet and lifestyle each day.

DISCRETIONARY CALORIES

(A new concept first described by the 2005 Dietary Guidelines Advisory Committee)

Discretionary calories = Total estimated energy requirements – Essential calories

When all food choices are in "nutrient-dense forms" that is lean or low-fat, with no added sugars then nutrient needs can be met with fewer calories than the amount required for energy balance. The calories needed to meet nutrient needs are called "essential calories." By subtracting the essential calories from a person's total energy requirements, the number of calories available for discretionary food choices can be determined. This remaining balance of discretionary calories permits some choices of foods with higher levels of fat and some added sugars intake, or increased intake from any food group. These amounts of "extras" however are lower than most Americans now consume.

As energy requirements increase with increased physical activity, the amount of discretionary calories increases.

Weight Management

If you are significantly overweight, you have a greater risk of developing many diseases, including high blood pressure, type 2 diabetes, stroke, and some forms of cancer. For obese adults, even losing a few pounds or preventing further weight gain has health benefits. Reaching a healthier weight is a balancing act. The secret is learning how to balance your "energy in" and "energy out" over the long run. "Energy in" is the calories from the foods and beverages you have each day. "Energy out" is the calories that you burn for basic body functions and physical activity.

Energy In = Energy Out

Your weight will stay the same when the calories that you eat and drink equal the calories that you burn.

Energy In < Energy Out

You will lose weight when the calories that you eat and drink are less than the calories that you burn.

Energy In > Energy Out

You will gain weight when the calories that you eat and drink are greater than the calories that you burn.

Physical Activity

For health benefits, physical activity should be **moderate** or **vigorous** and add up to at least 30 minutes a day. Everyone should get a minimum of 30 to 60 minutes each day of moderate exercise, brisk walking or bicycling, for example. Losing weight will require 60 to 90 minutes of more intense daily exercise.

Moderate Physical Activities Include:
- Walking briskly (about 3½ miles per hour)
- Hiking
- Gardening/yard work
- Dancing
- Golf (walking and carrying clubs)
- Bicycling (less than 10 miles per hour)
- Weight training (general light workout)

Vigorous Physical Activities Include:
- Running/jogging (5 miles per hour)
- Bicycling (more than 10 miles per hour)
- Swimming (freestyle laps)
- Aerobics
- Walking very fast (4½ miles per hour)
- Heavy yard work, such as chopping wood
- Weight lifting (vigorous effort)
- Competitive basketball

Food Groups to Encourage:
- Eat fruits and vegetables for a total of at least 4.5 cups (9 servings) each day
- Choose low-fat or fat-free milk, yogurt, and other dairy products
- Try to eat at least half of your grains as whole grain foods, or about 3 ounce-equivalents each day

What Counts as One Serving?

The amount of food that counts as one serving is listed in the following table.

Be sure to eat at least the lowest number of servings from the five major food groups listed. You need them for the vitamins, minerals, carbohydrates, and protein that they provide. Just try to pick the lowest fat choices from the food groups. No specific serving size is given for the fats, oils, and sweets group because the message is use sparingly.

Protein
- Go lean with protein.
- Consider dry beans and peas as an alternative to meat or poultry.
- Keep the overall amounts of foods eaten from this group within the amount needed each day. For example, people who need 2,000 calories per day need 5½ ounce-equivalents per day.

Milk, Yogurt, and Cheese		
1 cup of milk or yogurt	1½ ounces of natural cheese	2 ounces of process cheese

Meat, Poultry, Fish, Dry Beans, Eggs, and Nuts		
2 to 3 ounces of cooked lean meat, poultry, or fish	½ cup of cooked dry beans, 1 egg, or 2 tablespoons of peanut butter count as 1 ounce of lean meat	

Vegetable		
1 cup of raw leafy vegetables	½ cup of other vegetables, cooked or chopped raw	¾ cup of vegetable juice

Fruit		
1 medium apple, banana, orange	½ cup of chopped, cooked, or canned fruit	¾ cup of fruit juice

Bread, Cereal, Rice, and Pasta		
1 slice of bread	1 ounce of ready-to-eat cereal	½ cup of cooked cereal, rice, or pasta

Strategies for Protein

- Select meat cuts that are low in fat and ground beef that is extra lean (at least 90% lean).
- Trim fat from meat and removing poultry skin before cooking or eating.
- Drain fat from ground meats after cooking.
- Use preparation methods that do not add fat, such as grilling, broiling, poaching, or roasting.
- Choose lean turkey, roast beef, or ham or low-fat luncheon meats for sandwiches instead of fatty luncheon meats such as bologna or salami.

Consume a sufficient amount of fruits and vegetables while staying within your energy needs. Fruits and vegetables have a strong boost. Nine servings of produce are recommended for the average 2,000-calorie diet, which translates to 2 cups of fruit and 2½ cups of vegetables each day. Within the recommended 2 cups of fruit a day, whole fruit whether fresh, canned, frozen or dried is recommended rather than fruit juice to obtain an adequate amount of fiber.

Within the recommended 2½ cups of vegetables a day and whether you choose fresh, canned, or frozen you should include a variety from the following five subgroups throughout the week: dark green vegetables (spinach, most greens), legumes (dry beans, chickpeas), starchy vegetables (corn, green peas), orange vegetables (carrots, sweet potatoes), and other vegetables (tomatoes, green beans).

Strategies for Meeting Fruit Recommendation

- Use fruit in salads, toppings, desserts, and/or snacks regularly.
- Use fruit as a topping on cereal, pancakes, and other foods rather than sugars, syrups, or other sweet toppings.
- Select fruits that are in season to increase variety.
- Use canned, frozen, and dried fruits as well as fresh fruits.
- Avoid fruit canned in syrup. Light or heavy syrup adds sugar to canned fruits. Fruits canned in juice or water are a better choice.

Strategies for Vegetables

- Include vegetables in lunch, dinner, and snacks.
- Prepare main dishes, side dishes, and salads that include vegetables.
- Add vegetables to mixed dishes such as soups, stews, casseroles, and stir-fries.
- Add dark-green or orange vegetables to soups, stews, casseroles, and stir-fries.
- Use romaine, spinach, or other dark leafy greens as salad greens, and eat green salads often.
- Choose main dishes, side dishes, and salads that include cooked dry beans or peas.

Milk, Yogurt, and Cheese

Calcium builds strong bones to last a lifetime, so you need these foods in your diet. Choose fat-free or low-fat milk, yogurt, and cheese. If you choose milk or yogurt that is not fat-free, or cheese that is not low-fat, the fat in the product counts as part of the discretionary calorie allowance. If you choose sweetened milk products, e.g., flavored milk, yogurt, drinkable yogurt, desserts, you must count the added sugars as part of the discretionary calorie allowance.

For those who are lactose intolerant, lactose-free and lower-lactose products are available. Also, enzyme preparations can be added to milk to lower the lactose content.

Fats

Less than 10 percent of calories should come from saturated fats, and fat should make up no more than 25 to 30 percent of total calories. No firm guideline was set for trans fats, only a recommendation to keep them "as low as possible." The best sources should come from mainly polyunsaturated and monounsaturated fats: fish, nuts, vegetable oils.

Types of Fats

Saturated

- Meat
- Egg yolk
- Butter
- Dairy
- Coconut
- Palm oil

Polyunsaturated

- Vegetable oils
- Fish (omega-3s)
- Walnuts
- Almonds

Monounsaturated

- Olive oil
- Peanut oil
- Avocados

Trans Fats
- Labeled as "partially hydrogenated"

Strategies for Using Fats
- Choose "healthy fats" such as olive oil and canola oil.
- Use canola margarine and cook with canola oil.
- Use olive oil salad dressings.
- Avoid "unhealthy fats" such as saturated and trans fat.
- Check nutrition labels and ingredient lists.
- Choose low-fat dairy products and lean meats.
- Eat at least two seafood meals each week.
- Include a source of omega-3 fats.

Carbohydrates

The health benefits of eating whole grains include lowering the risk of:

- Coronary heart disease
- Type 2 diabetes
- Colon cancer
- Obesity

What Is a Whole Grain?
- Foods made with the entire grain seed (kernel).
- FDA health claim: Whole grain food must contain 51 percent or more whole grain ingredients by weight per reference amount and be low in fat and cholesterol.
- *Refined grains* have been milled, i.e., the bran and germ are removed. This process also removes much of the B vitamins, iron, and dietary fiber. Some refined grains are enriched. This means certain B vitamins (thiamin, riboflavin, niacin, folic acid) and iron are added back after processing. Fiber is not added back to most enriched grains.

Finding Whole Grains When Shopping

Good Source	A half serving (8g) of whole grain
Excellent Source	A full serving (16g) of whole grain
100%/Excellent	A full serving (16g) and all grains are whole

Examples of Whole Grains
- Amaranth
- Barley
- Brown rice
- Buckwheat
- Bulgur
- Kamut
- Millet
- Oatmeal
- Popcorn

- Quinoa
- Sorghum
- Spelt
- Whole corn
- Whole-grain pasta
- Whole rye
- Whole wheat
- Whole-wheat couscous
- Wild rice

Strategies for Consuming Carbohydrates
- Choose fiber-rich fruits, vegetables, and whole grains often.
- Choose and prepare foods and beverages with little added sugars or caloric sweeteners.
- Reduce the incidence of dental caries by consuming sugar- and starch-containing foods and beverages less frequently.
- Eat three or more ounce-equivalents of whole grain products per day.
- Half your grains should come from whole grains.

Sodium and Potassium
- Choose and prepare foods with little salt.
- Consume less than 2,300 mg (1 tsp salt) of sodium each day.
- Check food labels for sodium. Foods with less than 140 mg sodium (5% DV) are low in salt.

Consume Potassium-Rich Foods, Such as Fruits and Vegetables
- Some vegetables that are rich in potassium include sweet potatoes, beet greens, white potatoes, white beans, tomato products, soybeans, lima beans, winter squash, spinach, lentils, kidney beans, and split peas.
- Some fruits that are rich in potassium include prune juice, bananas, cantaloupe, honeydew, prunes, dried peaches or apricots, orange juice, and plantains. Some fruit juices, such as orange and prune juice, are rich in potassium.

Strategies for Sodium
- Beware that processed meats and fresh chicken, turkey, and pork that have been enhanced with a salt-containing solution also have added sodium.
- Beware that frozen dinners, packaged mixes, cereals, cheese, breads, soups, salad dressings, pickles, ketchup, olives, and sauces have added sodium.
- Beware that foods with less than 140 mg sodium per serving can be labeled as "low sodium foods."

Food Guide Pyramid for Kids Ages 4 to 13
Grains
- 4- to 8-year-olds need 4 to 5 ounce equivalents each day.
- 9- to 13-year-old girls need 5 ounce equivalents each day.
- 9- to 13-year-old boys need 6 ounce equivalents each day.

Vegetables

- 4- to 8-year-olds need 1½ cups of vegetables each day.
- 9- to 13-year-old girls need 2 cups of vegetables each day.
- 9- to 13-year-old boys need 2½ cups of vegetables each day.

Fruits

- 4- to 8-year-olds need 1– to 1½ cups of fruit each day.
- 9- to 13-year-olds need 1½ cups of fruit each day.

Milk and Other Calcium-Rich Foods

- 4- to 8-year-olds need 2 cups of milk (or another calcium-rich food) each day.
- 9- to 13-year-olds need 3 cups of milk (or another calcium-rich food) each day.

Meats, Beans, Fish, and Nuts

- 4- to 8-year-olds need 3 to 4 ounce equivalents each day.
- 9- to 13-year-olds need 5 ounce equivalents each day.

USDA PROPOSES NEW 2010 DIETARY GUIDELINES FOR AMERICANS

The new *2010 Advisory Committee report* observations are the following: "The single most significant adverse health trend among U.S. children in the past 40 years has been the dramatic increase in overweight and obesity. Since the early 1970s, the prevalence of overweight and obese people has approximately doubled among children ages 2 to 11 years, and tripled among adolescents' ages 12 to 19 years. Not only is obesity associated with adverse health effects during childhood, but evidence documents increased risk of future chronic disease in adult life."

The new guidelines can be shortly summarized with the following statements:

a) Eating a healthy balance of nutritious (nutrient dense) foods continues as a central point in the dietary guidelines, but balancing nutrients is not enough for health.

b) There is an emphasis on increased availability of fresh produce for consumers.

c) To place a stronger emphasis on calorie control and physical activity. The amount of total calories also should be considered.

d) Reduction of salt intake by 40%. The new guidelines lower the recommended maximum daily intake of salt from 2,300 milligrams to 1,500 milligrams.

e) General reduction of solid fats and added sugar (sugary foods and drinks).

f) To give preference on plant (vegetables and fruits) based diet.

g) To select a low fat, high on fiber, dairy and whole grains-based diet.

h) The improvement in nutrition based on cooking skills and home-cooked healthy foods and on creating new nutrition programs and physical education in schools.

(Source, *usda.gov*)

Specifically, the new 2010 dietary guidelines, which were released on January 31, 2011, aim for the following:

1. **Manage Calories to Manage Your Weight**
   - Balance calories and physical activity
   - Focus on nutrient-dense foods and drinks like whole grains, fruits, vegetables, healthy fats, and lean protein, as well as non-fat milk
   - For those already overweight or obese, the goal is to prevent further weight gain and encourage weight loss.

How is this different from the 2005 Guidelines?

Maintaining a healthy weight, reducing overweight and obesity are now major themes.

2. **What Foods to Reduce**
   - Focus on nutrient-dense foods and limit empty calorie foods
   - Limit sodium intake to less than 2,300 mg and to 1,500 mg for certain populations, i.e., African Americans
   - Limit calories from solid fats like butter
   - Limit added sugars like those found in sodas and other processed foods

How is this different from the 2005 Guidelines?

Limiting calories from added sugars and solid fats replaces the concept of discretionary calories.

3. **Foods and Nutrients to Increase**
   - Whole grains: at least half of grains consumed should be whole refined grain consumption.
   - Look for the word "whole" when purchasing grains
   - Protein: Increase fish and seafood consumption as well as plant-based sources of protein like legumes

How is this different from the 2005 Guidelines?

The whole grain recommendations continue to be the same for 2010, and for protein, the change is on increased variety of protein food sources consumed.

4. **Nutrients of Concern**
   - Americans are falling short in areas such as fiber intake, vitamin D, and calcium, as well as potassium. This is the result of a poor intake of produce and whole grains, as well as sources of non-fat dairy.

How is this different from the 2005 Guidelines?

Nutrients of concern reflect poor intake of key food sources rather than particular nutrients.

MY PLATE

As of press time for the edition, the USDA has developed a new good guide replacing the decades-old "my pyramid." It is called, "My Plate." It can be accessed at *www.choosemyplate.gov*

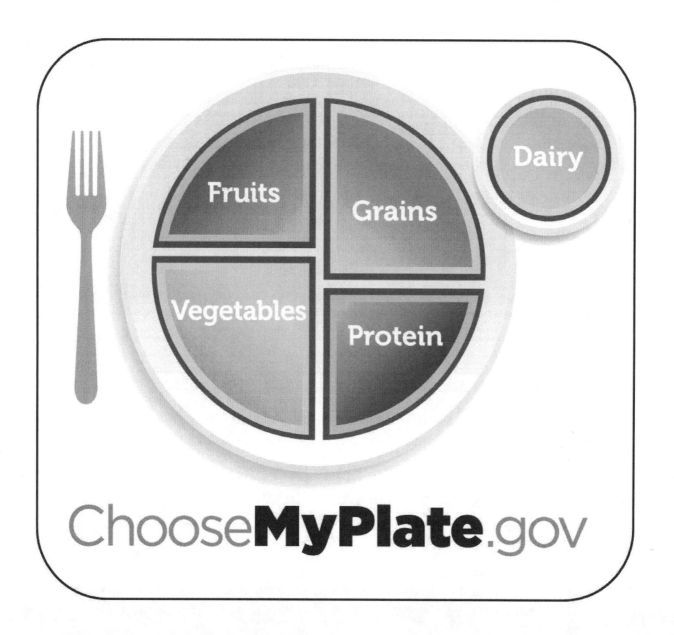

What's unique about this graphic is that it clearly divides a standard plate with foods and amounts that should be consumed. In other words, only one quarter of the plate should be filled with protein based foods. This is important since many Americans rely on fatty protein sources like beef, and other processed meats like bologna and pepperoni. This leaves the remaining three quarters of the plate coming from plant based food sources like fruits, vegetables and grains. It is a clear message to American consumers that a plant based diet fights disease and helps manage weight.

ASSIGNMENT #2

Go to *www.mypyramid.gov* and click on *mypyramid plan* and then *mypyramid menu planner*.

1. Enter your age, gender, and activity level to get your own plan at an appropriate calorie level. The food plan will include specific daily amounts from each food group and a limit for discretionary calories. Print out a personalized poster of your plan, and a worksheet to help you track your progress.

2. Describe your results, and compare it to your current eating habits.

    _____

    _____

    _____

    _____

    _____

    _____

    _____

    _____

    _____

    _____

    _____

3. What are some faults of the USDA's Food Pyramid?

    _____

    _____

    _____

    _____

    _____

    _____

    _____

    _____

    _____

4. List some tips for using the Harvard's Healthy Eating Pyramid.

_____

_____

_____

_____

_____

_____

_____

_____

_____

_____

_____

_____

RESOURCES

Buzby, J. C., Hodan, F. W., and Vocke, G. 2006. Possible Implications for U.S. Agriculture from Adoption of Select Dietary Guidelines. Economic Research Report No. ERR-31. *http://www.ers.usda.gov/Publications/ERR31/.*

Davis, C., Saltos, E. Dietary Recommendations and How They Have Changed Over Time. *http://www.ers.usda.gov/publications/aib750/aib750b.pdf*

Family Health Administration: *http://www.fha.state.md.us/ocd/cardio/html/eatingfacts.html.*

Food Pyramid image: *http://www.usda.gov/cnpp/pyramid.htm*

Harvard Nutritionist says USDA 'Food Pyramid' is Wrong: http://www.rense.com/general12/wrong.htm

www.healthierus.gov/dietaryguidelines

"MyPyramid.gov access point." 2005. United States Department of Agriculture. DGAC report, Part D. Science Base, Sect. 6. Selected Food Groups.

Reyes, R. 2008. "Food Pyramid Frenzy," *Wall Street Journal*, July 15. 2006–12.

Schlosberg, S., Neporent, L. 2005. *Fitness for Dummies*, 3rd ed. "For Dummies" (Wiley).

U.S. Department of Health and Human Services and U.S. Department of Agriculture. Dietary Guidelines for Americans. 2005. 6th ed. Washington, DC: U.S. Government Printing Office. Available at: *http://www.mypyramid.gov/guidelines/index.html*

U.S. Department of Agriculture. MyPyramid. 2005. *http://www.pyramid.gov.*

Willet, W. 2005. *Eat, Drink and Be Healthy: The Harvard Medical School Guide to Healthy Eating.* Simon & Schuster.

chapter 3
The Nutrients

Nutrients are what keep us alive; they are our building blocks. Nutrients are substances found in food that help promote the growth and maintenance of our bodies. There are six essential nutrients. Remember, "essential" here means that our body cannot make them on its own, and, therefore, must obtain them through food. They are:

1. Carbohydrates
2. Lipids (chemical name for a family of fatty substances)
3. Protein
4. Vitamins
5. Minerals
6. Water

CARBOHYDRATES

Carbohydrates were discovered through the early investigations of chemists. By pouring sugar into test tubes and then burning it over a heat source, they saw that two major products were formed: water and a black substance called carbon. Thus, the name carbo (think: carbon) hydrate (think: water) was determined. The main elements making up carbohydrates are carbon, hydrogen, and oxygen. Carbohydrates are found mostly in plant-based foods. Plants are able to make their own carbohydrates through a process known as photosynthesis. Photosynthesis converts energy from the sun into energy stored in carbohydrates, which the plant uses to grow. Animals are incapable of photosynthesis and must get carbohydrates from plant-based foods like wheat, corn, fruits, and other vegetables. In other words, when eating bread, rice, cereal, pasta, or an apple, or broccoli, you are eating a carbohydrate.

Carbohydrates are the body's preferred energy source. In fact, they are so important, the body's central nervous system, which is composed of the brain and spine, functions solely off of carbohydrates. In other words, carbohydrates are brain fuel!

By now, almost everyone has heard of the Atkins Diet (*Doctor Atkins' New Diet Revolution*, 1999), which promotes weight loss through the consumption of foods low in carbohydrates and quite high in fat and protein contents, but not necessarily low in calories.

How Do These Diets Work?

You have learned that carbohydrates are crucial to central nervous system function. So, how is it that someone can consume a no-carbohydrate diet, like the Atkins Diet? By drastically restricting carbohydrate consumption, the body goes into a different metabolic state called ketosis, where it burns its own fat and protein for fuel. When the body doesn't receive carbohydrates from its daily diet, it will start to burn protein, which is capable of being converted into a useable form of glucose (carbohydrate) to provide energy to the central nervous system. Meanwhile, fat is burned to feed other tissues and organs. However, a byproduct called ketones is produced when fat is burned without the presence of carbohydrates. This is not good! A person in ketosis is getting energy from ketones which are little carbon fragments that are the fuel created by the breakdown of fat stores. When the body is in ketosis, you tend to feel less hungry, and, as a result, you are likely to eat less than you might otherwise. Ketosis can also cause the following health problems:

Kidney Failure

Consuming too much protein puts a strain on the kidneys, which can make a person susceptible to kidney disease.

High Cholesterol

High-protein diets are typically also high in saturated fat and dietary cholesterol (consisting of red meat, whole dairy products, and other high fat foods). This type of diet is linked to high cholesterol. Studies have linked high cholesterol levels to an increased risk of developing heart disease, stroke, and cancer.

Osteoporosis and Kidney Stones

High-protein diets have been shown to cause people to excrete more calcium than normal through their urine. Over a prolonged period of time, this can increase a person's risk of osteoporosis and kidney stones.

Cancer

One of the reasons high-protein diets may increase the risks of certain health problems is because of the avoidance of carbohydrate-containing foods and the vitamins, minerals, fiber, and antioxidants they contain. It is, therefore, important to obtain your protein from a diet rich in whole grains, legumes, nuts, and low-fat dairy. Not only are you meeting your protein needs, but you are also helping to reduce your risk of developing cancer.

Ketosis

Low-carbohydrate diets can cause your body to go into a dangerous metabolic state called ketosis because your body burns fat instead of glucose for energy. During ketosis, the body forms substances known as ketones, which can cause organs to fail and result in gout, kidney stones, or kidney failure. Ketones can also dull a person's appetite, and cause nausea and bad breath. Ketosis can be prevented by eating at least 100 grams of carbohydrates a day.

In 2003 (Foster et al.), a landmark study was reported in the *New England Journal of Medicine*. The researchers conducted a controlled experiment to determine the differences in weight loss of both obese men and women who consumed either the basic low-carbohydrate Atkins Diet or a conventional diet of reduced total calories. The study lasted for one year. After three months, the volunteers who ate the Atkins Diet lost 7 to 10 percent of their original body weight, while those who ate the conventional low-calorie diet only lost 3 to 5 percent of their original weight. After six months, the results were similar to those at three months; ***however,*** after one year, those on the Atkins Diet had regained enough weight so that differences in weight loss between the two diets were not significant.

CARBOHYDRATE TYPES

Not all carbohydrates are created equal. Some are good for health, and some are bad and, therefore, should be limited.

There are two main categories of carbohydrates:

1. Simple
2. Complex

Simple Carbohydrates

Simple carbohydrates can be *defined* as:

Added and natural sugars

Added Sugars

Let's take a closer look at what foods contain added sugars. Added sugars are found primarily in processed foods, such as cookies, cakes, candies, sugared cereals, and sodas. In fact, most Americans are consuming more added sugar than ever before.

A United States Department of Agriculture (USDA) survey showed that sugar consumption has increased almost every year since 1982. Much of the increase is due to the consumption of soft drinks (CSPI, 1999).

The USDA advises people who eat a 2,000-calorie diet to try to limit themselves to about 10 teaspoons of added sugars per day. In fact, the average American consumes roughly 20 teaspoons of added sugars per day. Below are some examples of sugar content for common foods:

- 1 typical cup of fruit yogurt provides 70% of a day's worth of added sugar
- 1 cup of regular ice cream provides 60%
- 1 12-ounce Pepsi provides 103%
- 1 Hostess Lemon Fruit Pie provides 115%
- 1 serving of Kellogg's Marshmallow Blasted *Froot Loops* provides 40%
- 1 quarter-cup of pancake syrup provides 103%

Natural Sugars

Natural sugars are those found in nature. They are found in two predominant foods: fruits and dairy.

Now that we have defined simple carbohydrates (added and natural sugars), let's take a closer look at the two categories of sugars:

1. Monosaccharides

2. Disaccharides

Sugars are either a one-unit (mono) sugar or a two-unit (di) sugar. There are three **monosaccharides:**

1. *Glucose*—Most simple of all sugars, major sugar found in the blood

2. *Fructose*—Fruit sugar

3. *Galactose*—Seldom found free in nature, part of lactose, the sugar found in milk

There are three **disaccharides,** and they each contain a glucose.

1. Glucose + Glucose = *Maltose*—sugar produced whenever starch breaks down, such as in beer production

2. Glucose + Fructose = *Sucrose*—table sugar

3. Glucose + Galactose = *Lactose*—Milk sugar

It is important to recognize at this point that *both* added and natural sugars contain the same amount of calories per gram (4) because they are both types of carbohydrates. In other words, your body does *not* distinguish between the sugar in a lollipop (added) and the sugar in an apple (natural). You might then ask, *Why do I have to limit my consumption of added sugars then?* The answer is simple: foods rich in natural sugars contain many other nutrients, like fiber, vitamins, and minerals that foods with a lot of added sugars typically do not contain. At the end of the day, a sugar is a sugar is a sugar.

For example, many people think honey is better for you than regular table sugar. Not so fast. Let's look at their chemical composition.

Table Sugar	vs.	*Honey*
Glucose + Fructose		Glucose + Fructose

They're the same thing! In fact, 1 teaspoon of sugar (the amount in a packet you'd get at Starbucks or Dunkin' Donuts) contains 16 calories, or 4g of carbohydrate. One teaspoon of honey, depending on the brand, contain anywhere from 25 to 40 calories! Why? Honey is highly concentrated. So, if someone is trying to lose weight, a packet of sugar at 16 calories would be preferable to a teaspoon of honey.

COMPLEX CARBOHYDRATES

The opposite of "simple" is "complex." Complex carbohydrates are said to be "complicated" in their chemical composition. In other words, think of a simple carbohydrate as looking like a simple wedding ring. And think of a complex carbohydrate looking like a chain-link necklace.

Two main types of complex carbohydrates exist:

1. *Starch:* Starch is defined as long chains of glucoses (monosaccharide) strung together, like the chains on a necklace.

2. *Fiber:* The indigestible portion of the plant foods that we eat.

Let's first discuss starch. Starch is technically part of a grain. There are many different types of grains such as wheat, corn, rice, barley, and oats to name a few. Grains contain three component parts with each part containing something specific. Think of an ear of corn. Now, imagine one of the kernels. This is a grain and it contains:

1. **Germ**—Tiny part of the grain containing trace amounts of oil and some vitamins and minerals. The germ is what is pressed when making some oils. For example, it takes 14 ears of corn to make 1 tablespoon of corn oil.

2. **Bran**—Rich in fiber, vitamins, and minerals.

3. **Endosperm**—Contains starch, and a little protein.

When these three component parts are intact, the grain is referred to as a *whole grain*. Have you heard that you should try to eat more whole grains? The reason is because these grains are rich in fiber, vitamins, and minerals. Unfortunately, the grains Americans consume most are referred to as, "refined." A *refined grain* contains only the endosperm; the germ and the bran have been removed during processing. What has been lost as a result? Fiber, vitamins, and minerals. In fact, a total of 22 vitamins and minerals are lost during processing.

Refined grains had a profound health impact on American health during the Great Depression. Since most people during this time struggled to afford basic necessities like food, many relied on government supplied subsidies, which included refined flour. Eating little else, many Americans began to develop deficiency diseases as a result. In an effort to solve this problem, the federal government required all refined grains to be *enriched*. An enriched grain is one that has some nutrients lost during processing replaced afterward. In this case, the most important vitamins and minerals were put back. In fact, even today, it is the law that all refined grains contain the following four vitamins and one mineral. Take a closer look at the ingredient's list of your next food purchase. See if you can find these nutrients.

1. Folic Acid

2. Niacin

3. Thiamin

4. Riboflavin

5. Iron (only mineral)

WHY REFINE?

Clearly, whole grains are better for health compared to refined grains. Even though some of the lost vitamins and minerals are replaced, fiber is not replaced. You may be wondering at this point, if whole grains are so much healthier for you than refined grain, why are they refined in the first place? There are three main reasons:

1. *Longer shelf life:* Because whole grains contain a trace amount of oil, they can become rancid (spoil or rot) fairly quickly. That's why it is important to store whole grain breads in the refrigerator rather than on countertops.

2. *Profits:* A company can make more money when it breaks apart a grain. The bran can be sold as "bran flakes" cereal. The oil can be pressed into, say, corn oil. The germ can be sold as wheat germ. All of this adds up to more revenue for companies.

3. *Taste:* Most Americans are accustomed to the taste of refined grains, which make products that are fluffier and doughier in taste. Whole grains make a nuttier, denser product.

BUYING WHOLE GRAINS

Finding and shopping for whole grains can be tricky. Here are some rules:

*   Don't use a product's color as a guide. In other words, don't assume just because a loaf of bread is brown that it is automatically a whole grain.

- Look for the word *whole* on the package. It must say "whole" in order to be a true whole grain. For example, "100% natural stone ground wheat bread" is NOT a whole grain; however, "100% natural stone ground whole wheat bread" is.
- For rice only, you must see the word *brown*. For example, "basmati rice" is not a whole grain, but "brown basmati rice" is.
- Oats and corn are rarely refined, so even if you do not see the word whole, you can be confident that you are eating a whole grain.

Now that we've discussed starch, let's take a closer look at fiber, our second complex carbohydrate.

FIBER

Fiber is the indigestible portion of the plant foods we eat. No animal-based products contain fiber.
There are two main types of fiber:

1. *Soluble fiber*

2. *Insoluble fiber*

The term *soluble* refers to something's ability to dissolve in water. So, soluble fiber does dissolve in water while insoluble does not.

All plant foods contain *both* types of fiber. Some foods, however, contain higher amounts of one type vs. the other.

Soluble fiber binds with fatty substances in your body and helps promote their excretion as waste, thereby lowering cholesterol levels. Some foods particularly rich in soluble fiber include oats (like oatmeal), sweet potatoes, berries (like strawberries and raspberries), and legumes.

Insoluble fiber adds bulk to your fecal matter, thereby speeding up the rate of your bowel movements. Foods particularly rich in insoluble fiber include corn and other whole grains.

Most Americans have no idea how many grams of fiber they get from their daily diets. Yet, for many people, this number should be doubled.

A recent American Dietetic Association position paper (Marlett et al., 2002) reported that most Americans do not even come close to the recommended intake of 20 to 35 grams of fiber a day. Americans' mean fiber intake is about half that, about 14–15 grams a day. Children should consume their age plus 5g of fiber. So, a 5-year-old should consume 10g of fiber per day (5 years old + 5 = 10g).

The amount of carbohydrate from starch and sugars that you should consume each day varies widely depending on your activity levels and goals. The 2005 Dietary Reference Intake report established acceptable macronutrient distribution ranges (AMDR) for carbohydrate. Adults and children (over 1 year old) should obtain 45 to 65 percent of their calories from carbohydrates. The wide range allows for more flexibility for people with various carbohydrate needs.

Fiber and Health: Diverticular Disease

Diverticular disease is a range of conditions caused by small pouches called diverticula along the colon wall. Once these pouches develop, a person is said to have diverticulosis. Diverticulitis is a more serious form of the disease where the diverticula become inflamed and infected. Women and men are equally affected.

While experts are not 100% certain as to what causes diverticulosis, weakened muscles along the colon wall as well as a low fiber diet are thought to be factors. Lack of physical activity, and overweight/obesity are also thought to be contributors. Diverticular disease is rare in areas of the world such as rural Africa and Asia where diets high in roughage, including high fiber grains as well as low consumption of red meat and fats are common.

People with diverticulosis often don't have any symptoms though some patients report abdominal cramping and bloating. Treatment includes medications, increase in fiber intake, physical activity, and water. Surgery is required in severe cases of diverticulitis where complications such as perforation of the colon, infection of the abdominal cavity, bowel obstruction, abscess and fistula—where there is an abnormal connection between the colon and nearby tissue—occur.

LIPIDS

Lipid is the chemical name for a family of fatty substances. There are several types of lipids such as saturated, unsaturated, and cholesterol. It is very important to understand that these are all *members* of the same family; they are not, however, all the same thing. Do not confuse saturated fat with, say, cholesterol. That would be like saying your brother or sister is the same as you because you come from the same family.

Saturated Fats

Like carbohydrates, lipids are made of carbon, hydrogen, and oxygen.

Saturated fats, however, are saturated, or filled to capacity, with hydrogens. This saturation with hydrogens is what makes consuming a lot of saturated fat bad for your blood vessels and overall health.

The general rule of thumb regarding saturated fats is that they typically come from animal-based foods with the exception of coconut and palm oils, which are plant-based, and often referred to as "tropical oils." Also, they are typically solid at room temperature. If you leave a stick of butter on the kitchen counter overnight, you will find the next day that it is not a liquid! It is still a solid. It is softer, but still solid.

Let's look at the food pyramid to identify where we might find a lot of saturated fat.

Bread, rice, cereal, and pasta are rich in carbohydrate and some fiber. In fact, although many people think these foods are "fattening," the reality is that they are either very low in fat or nonfat. It's not until someone adds cream cheese to a bagel, or butter to some rice or, alfredo sauce to some pasta that these foods then become fattening. Alone, however, they are very low in fat.

All fruits, with the exception of the avocado, which is technically a fruit though it is used as a vegetable in the United States, are fat-free or extremely low in fat.

All vegetables, with the exception of olives, which are pressed to make olive oil, are fat-free or extremely low in fat.

Dairy products can either be whole (full fat), low-fat, or nonfat. It is important to read food labels when shopping to ensure that you buy the lowest fat version available. For example, milk in the dairy aisle can be purchased as whole milk (usually has a red cap), low-fat (usually has a yellow cap), or nonfat (usually has a blue cap). Cheeses can also be purchased as full fat, low-fat, or nonfat. Ultimately, dairy can either be very high fat or virtually fat-free.

Meats can contain high amounts of saturated fat. Beef is like dairy in that you can purchase cuts that are high in fat or cuts that are lower in fat. Usually, cuts ending in "loin," such as sirloin or tenderloin are quite lean. Flank steak, fillet mignon, top or bottom rounds are also quite lean. Stay away from T-bone steaks, porterhouse, or other cuts with visible marbling. Marbling on a cut of steak or ground beef (the white streaks or specks you see) is all saturated fat. Chicken is quite low in fat, just avoid the skin, which is all saturated fat. White meat has less saturated fat than dark meat, however, dark meat is richer in the mineral iron than white meat. Pork can be quite lean or fatty. Bacon, sausage, and salami are all very high in saturated fat. Pork tenderloin, however, is very lean. Whatever the meat, be sure to look for fatty streaks or marbling. The more you see, the higher the saturated fat.

Beans (legumes) are very low in saturated fat. Nuts, on the other hand, are high in fat, but not saturated (see the rule above).

All seafood is fairly low in saturated fat. People find this hard to believe mostly because they associated seafood with deep frying. If you dip lobster into butter or fry shrimp in lard, it does become rich in saturated fat. But, on its own, it is quite low in saturated fat.

Unsaturated Fats

The general rule of thumb regarding unsaturated fats is that they typically come from plant-based foods with the exception of seafood, which are animal-based. Also, they are typically liquid at room temperature, like olive oil. Unsaturated fats are always preferable to saturated fats because they do not clog arteries like saturated fats do.

There are two types of unsaturated fats:

1. *Monounsaturated*—This type has one (mono) point of unsaturation (making it preferable to health). It helps increase "good" levels of blood cholesterol. Foods and oils rich in monounsaturated fats include avocado, peanuts, almonds, olive oil, canola oil, peanut oil, and nut butters like peanut or almond butter.

2. *Polyunsaturated*—This type has more than one (poly) point of unsaturation (making it preferable to health). There are two types of polyunsaturated fats:
   * Linoleic fatty acid (sometimes referred to as omega-6 fatty acid): This type of polyunsaturated fat increases inflammation and blood clotting in the body. Foods and oils rich in this type of lipid include vegetable oil (which is really soybean oil), corn oil, safflower oil, sunflower oil, cottonseed oil.
   * Linolenic fatty acid (sometimes referred to as omega-3 fatty acid): This type of polyunsaturated fat decreases inflammation and blood clotting in the body. Foods and oils rich in this type of lipid include seafood especially fatty fish like tuna, salmon, halibut, and bluefish; flaxseed, tofu, and walnuts.

Note that linoleic and linolenic fatty acids act as antagonists with each other. It is best to have a *balance* of both types in your diet. The reason you may have heard that Americans should try to consume more fatty fish in their diets is because the typical American diet is especially rich in linoleic fatty acids. To balance that out, it is a good idea to eat foods rich in linolenic fatty acids, like fatty fish or other source,s several times per week.

A key to understanding the different fats is remembering that whether they are good or bad for health, 1 gram of lipid contains 9 calories. In other words, do not go crazy eating "healthy" fats; they are still very high in calories!

Cholesterol

Cholesterol is a waxy substance that is often demonized, but it actually is crucial for all cellular functions in the body. It also is a key ingredient in the making of bile, which helps digest other lipids.

What is unique about cholesterol is that it is found *only in animal products*. That is because cholesterol is produced by the liver, and only animals (not plants!) have a liver. So, would peanut butter contain dietary cholesterol? Peanuts are plant-based. It is high in cholesterol's cousin, monounsaturated fat, but not cholesterol.

What is important to understand about cholesterol is that there is cholesterol we get from the foods we eat, called *dietary cholesterol*. Then, there is cholesterol that our liver produces on its own, which is often referred to as *blood serum cholesterol*. This is what your doctor measures to determine if you have high cholesterol or not. Many people still believe that eating foods high in dietary cholesterol (i.e., eggs, shrimp) are what cause you to have high blood serum cholesterol. We now know that its effect is not as strong as that of saturated fats or trans fats (DeBruyne, Pinna & Whitney, 2008).

Typically, doctors look for total cholesterol to be under 200mg/dL. Yet, we all hear about the person whose cholesterol is "normal" who has a heart attack. What is going on?

"Good" cholesterol, technically known as high density lipoprotein (HDL), is a type of cholesterol produced by the liver that helps unclog blood vessels. Eating an overall diet low in saturated and trans fats with an emphasis on unsaturated fats can help increase HDL. Vigorous exercise, as well as moderate alcohol consumption, may also help increase this good cholesterol (De Oliveira e Silva *et al.*, 2000).

"Bad" cholesterol, technically known as low density lipoprotein (LDL), is a type of cholesterol produced by the liver that clogs blood vessels. Eating a diet rich in saturated and trans fats stimulates the liver to make this type of cholesterol. Why?

The bloodstream is composed mostly of water. When we eat a fat, whether it is in saturated or unsaturated form, it must be absorbed into the bloodstream from the small intestine. Herein lies the problem. The fatty blob cannot move smoothly through our watery bloodstream. To solve this transit problem, the liver is called upon to secrete lipoproteins. If you eat a lot of bad-for-you saturated and trans fats, then your liver excretes a lot of "bad" LDL cholesterol to help its transport. On the other hand, if you consume a lot of unsaturated fats, the liver is stimulated to produce more of the "good" HDL cholesterol.

Back to the heart attack patient with "normal" total cholesterol. The problem is that many Americans have "normal" cholesterol, but have disproportionate levels of HDL and LDL. Having high LDL and low HDL may make your total cholesterol appear normal.

It is best to aim for an LDL number of less than 100mg/dL. And it is ideal to have an HDL of 60mg/dL or higher.

Trans Fats

Trans fats are a man-made lipid (although a small amount of the trans fat we eat is found naturally in animal foods) that was developed in the 1980s. Around this time, consumers were looking for foods lower in fat. In response, food companies developed trans fats, also known as partially hydrogenated fats, which, at the time, were understood to be a healthier alternative to artery-clogging saturated fats. The trans fats allowed foods to still taste creamy, flaky, and crispy.

We now know that a diet containing trans fats is very unhealthy. Like saturated fat, consumption of trans fats raises LDL cholesterol (so-called "bad cholesterol") increasing your risk of heart disease. Unlike saturated fat, however, trans fat is thought to lower HDL cholesterol (so-called "good cholesterol").

A trans fat is one that begins as a healthy, unsaturated fat. It then is "hydrogenated," whereby hydrogen atoms are pumped into it replacing some of the hydrogens it was originally missing.

Remember, it started off as an unsaturated fat. The result is a partially hydrogenated fat or trans fat. These fats are found primarily in processed foods. In January 2006, the Food and Drug Administration (FDA) required all packaged foods to disclose on the nutrition facts panel how many grams of trans fat the product contained. There is a slight loophole to this rule. A product can claim zero grams of trans fat *if* it contains less than 0.5 grams of trans fat per serving. Although that is a small amount of trans fat, if you eat multiple servings of foods with less than 0.5 grams of trans fat, you could exceed recommended limits. To be sure, read the ingredient's list. If you see the words *partially hydrogenated,* the product contains trans fat.

The recommended dietary allowance (RDA) for lipids is 30 percent of total calories. This 30 percent, however, should not be comprised of saturated fats. In fact, no more than 10 percent (of the 30 percent total) should come from saturated fats. Ideally, all 30 percent would come from unsaturated fat food sources. The American Heart Association (2002) recommends that no more than 1 percent of your total daily calories be trans fat. If you consume 2,000 calories a day, you should have no more than 2 grams of trans fat or less.

PROTEIN

Protein in food does not provide body proteins directly, but rather supply the amino acids from which the body makes its own proteins.

Protein is found in both animal- and vegetable-based foods. Animal sources include:

- Meats, like beef, pork, lamb
- Poultry, like chicken and turkey
- Dairy, like cheese, milk, and yogurt
- Seafood
- Eggs

It is also found in vegetable-based sources such as:

- Legumes, like black beans and kidney beans
- Nuts, like almonds and walnuts
- Grains, like wheat (remember the endosperm?)

Proteins are made of substances known as amino acids. You can think of amino acids as being like links in a chain necklace. They string together to form a protein. Twenty different amino acids exist (DeBruyne, Pinna & Whitney, 2008) and are divided into two groups: essential and nonessential.

There are 9 essential amino acids that the body cannot make on its own and must obtain through food. There are 11 nonessential amino acids that the body *can* make on its own. In fact, the body manufactures these amino acids from the essential amino acids. If a person fails to get the 9 essential amino acids in his or her diet, then the nonessential amino acids become essential. If this happens, the amino acid is said to be "conditionally essential."

High- and Low-Quality Proteins

High-quality proteins provide enough of all the essential amino acids needed to support the body's work, whereas low-quality proteins do not. To determine a protein's "quality," both its amino acid composition and digestibility are taken into account. Animal-based foods (meat, fish, poultry, dairy, and eggs) are considered high-quality protein sources and contain all of the essential amino acids. Protein derived from plant-based foods (legumes, nuts, and grains) tend to be limiting in one or more essential amino acids and, therefore, are considered low-quality protein sources. Soy protein, however, is one exception; it is high-quality protein just like that found in animal-based foods.

What happens if someone does not eat animal-based products? Vegans are the strictest types of vegetarians who consume *no* animal-based foods. To ensure that they are getting enough high-quality protein, they will either eat:

1. Soy-based products, such as tofu.

2. Complementary proteins, which are a combination of a grain and a legume, such as beans and rice. Each food supplies the amino acids missing in the other.

Often, when people think of protein, they think only of muscle building, but protein has other important bodily functions:

- Antibody production: Antibodies protect the body against bacteria, viruses, and other disease agents. Protein we eat helps build antibodies. In third world countries, where protein rich foods are scarce, sickness often occurs due to lack of antibody production.
- Hormone production: Protein helps build proteins, which are "chemical messengers" in the body. An example is the hormone insulin.
- Acid-base balance: Proteins also help maintain the balance between acids and bases within the body's fluids. Normal body processes constantly make acids and bases, which are carried by the bloodstream to the kidneys and lungs for excretion. The blood has to do this without upsetting the acid-base balance. Proteins act as buffers during this process helping to maintain the acid-base balance of the blood and body fluids.
- Enzyme production: Enzymes speed up chemical reactions. All enzymes are proteins. There are many different enzymes in the body that perform a range of tasks like digestion, for example.
- Growth, maintenance, and repair: The body is constantly building and repairing itself. Both inside and outside the body, cells constantly make and break down their proteins. People need to eat protein-rich foods daily to replace the protein they continually lose.

The recommended dietary allowance for protein for healthy adults is 0.8 gram per kilogram (2.2 pounds) of body weight. This results in roughly 10 to 35 percent of energy intake. For example:

1. Determine your body weight in pounds and then convert to kilograms (pounds divided by 2.2).

2. Multiply kilograms by 0.8 to determine total grams of protein recommended.

There are some populations that have higher-than-average protein requirements. In the United States, there is no shortage of protein in the daily diet. Yet, many people feel compelled to consume protein supplements. If too much protein is eaten, it can be stored as body fat. Also, extra protein burdens the kidneys. Athletes believe that protein shakes made with whey protein (a by-product of dairy manufacturing) will help their performance. Although whey protein may increase protein synthesis slightly, it does not appear to improve athletic performance (Tipton, 2004).

Periods of growth make protein consumption especially important for the following groups:

- Infants, children, and adolescents
- Pregnant or lactating women
- Physically active people

Protein Recommendations for Physically Active People:

Goal:	Grams/Kilograms
Strength train, maintain	1.0–1.2
Strength train, gain muscle mass	1.5–1.7
Moderate intensity endurance activities	1.2
High intensity endurance training	1.6

Source: Burke, L., Deakin, V., 2000.

VITAMINS AND MINERALS

Vitamins and minerals are found in foods in tiny quantities, much smaller than the energy-yielding nutrients. Vitamins and minerals contribute no energy to the body; instead, they assist the body with most of its processes.

Vitamins: A Timeline

1915: When widespread looting strips Shanghai, China, of food sources, Carnation businessman, Carl Rehnborg, develops the first food supplement: a combination of ground-up leaves, animal bones, and rusty nails for iron.

1927–1934: In California, Rehnborg markets a multivitamin named "Nutrilite."

1930s: Depression food shortages lead to significant nutrient deficiencies. Food manufacturers begin fortifying foods. Multivitamin makers are quick to get in on the action. By 1939, vitamin sales hit over $82 million.

1942: Vitamin sales reach over $130 million.

1968: USDA study reports that half of households do not consume the recommended dietary allowances of at least one vitamin or mineral. Vitamin companies use these findings in their marketing strategies.

1994: Under President Bill Clinton, the Dietary Supplement Health and Education Act removes supplements from the FDA's oversight, allowing manufacturers to make grand health claims. Sales total $4 billion.

2008: Consumers spend more than $25 billion annually on supplements. An estimated 35% of Americans take a multivitamin regularly.

Prevention magazine, November 2010

Vitamins fall into two categories:

1. Fat soluble

2. Water soluble

Fat-Soluble

The fat-soluble vitamins dissolve in fatty substances in the body, not water. Since there is an abundance of fatty tissue in the body, these types of vitamins are particularly worrisome if taken in megadoses. Instead of the excess being excreted, as happens with water-soluble vitamins, excess fat-soluble vitamins are stored in the body's fatty tissues.

There are four main fat-soluble vitamins: A, D, E, and K. To remember them, string the letters (A, D, E, K) together to form a word. ADEK sounds like the real word, *attic*, as in, you store your holiday decorations in the attic.

Vitamin A

- First fat-soluble vitamin to be recognized
- Helps overall eye health
- Prevents night blindness
- Beta-carotene: a vitamin A precursor (inactive forms of certain vitamins. Once inside the body, a precursor is converted to the active form of the vitamin). Also, an orange pigment found in fruits and vegetables like carrots.
- Acts as an antioxidant
- Good sources: fortified milk, carrots, sweet potatoes, liver, egg yolks

Antioxidants

The antioxidants are vitamins A, C, and E. String them together to help you remember them. They form the word, *ace*, like an ace bandage you would use to wrap a sprained ankle. Antioxidants act like police officers patrolling your body for substances called free radicals. Free radicals are substances that damage the body's cells. They are caused by exposure to pollutants, smoking, poor diet, and normal body processes. Antioxidants scour the body looking for these free radicals and promote their excretion as waste.

Vitamin D

- Sun exposure helps the body synthesize it on its own
- Helps the body absorb calcium important for bone health
- Good sources: egg yolks, liver, butter, some fatty fish, fortified milk

Vitamin E

- Acts as an antioxidant
- Good sources: vegetable oils, nuts, seeds

Vitamin K

- Helps with blood clotting
- Roughly 50 percent produced by bacteria in intestines
- Good sources: leafy greens like collard greens, and spinach, as well as vegetable oils like soy and canola

Water-Soluble

Water-soluble vitamins dissolve in the watery fluids of the body. Although it is difficult, it is still possible to mega-dose on these types of vitamins. Because they are water-soluble, any excess consumed is excreted through the urine as waste. That is why if you take a lot of vitamin C, for example, which is a water-soluble vitamin, you may notice that your urine is bright yellow. You are literally peeing away your money! The body excreted what it did not need. The following are the main water-soluble vitamins.

Vitamin C

- Acts as an antioxidant
- Prevents scurvy, a debilitating deficiency disease that causes gums to bleed, teeth to fall out, and eventual death. Sailors on long voyages were susceptible to scurvy after perishable fruits and vegetables were consumed. Once it was determined that citrus fruits helped prevent scurvy, sailors were given lime juice to help prevent it.
- Builds collagen, which helps give elasticity to skin, ligaments, and tendons
- Good sources: citrus fruits, bell peppers, broccoli, berries

Folate

- Activates vitamin B12
- Helps synthesize DNA for new cell growth (think of a growing baby)
- Helps prevent neural tube defects like spina bifida (which literally means *open spine*)
- Good sources: leafy greens, enriched grains, beans

Vitamin B12

- Found *only* in animal-based foods, except for fortified cereals
- Activates folate
- Protects nerve cells
- Good soruces: meat, poultry, fish, dairy, eggs, fortified cereals

Minerals

There are two categories of minerals: major and trace. The distinction between the major and trace minerals does not mean that one group is more important than the other. The major minerals, for example, are so named because they are needed in larger amounts by the body than the trace minerals.

Let's start with the *major minerals*.

Calcium

- Strengthens bones and teeth
- Aids muscle contraction
- Helps regulate blood pressure
- Good sources: dairy products, small fish with bones (sardines), greens like broccoli

The Electrolytes

Sodium, potassium, and chloride are major minerals also known as electrolytes. Electrolytes help maintain the body's fluid balance and its acid-base balance.

Sodium

- Good sources: salt, soy sauce, process foods. The American diet is too rich in sodium resulting in hypertension.

Potassium

- All whole foods like fruits and vegetables, milk, grains, beans, and meats.

Chloride

- In addition to functioning as an electrolyte, chloride is part of the hydrochloric acid enzyme found in the stomach.
- Good sources: salt, soy sauce, processed foods

Trace Minerals

Iron

- Part of the protein hemoglobin, which carries oxygen in the blood
- Anemia is the deficiency disease associated with lack of iron
- Good sources: red meats, fish, poultry, eggs, beans, dried fruits, spinach

Iodine

- Helps thyroid function, which plays a key role in metabolic regulation
- Good sources: iodized salt, seafood

Fluoride

- Helps make teeth resistant to decay that causes cavities
- Too much can cause fluorosis (discoloration of the teeth)
- Good sources: municipal water supplies that are fluoridated, some tea and seafood

WATER

The human body is composed of roughly 60 percent water making it an extremely vital nutrient. Every cell in the body is rich in fluid.

Functions of water in the body:

- Carries nutrients and wastes throughout the body
- Cushions and lubricates joints and bones
- Helps maintain blood pressure
- Helps maintain normal body temperature
- Helps maintain blood volume

Water intake is regulated by part of the brain known as the hypothalamus. When the blood becomes too concentrated, the mouth becomes dry and the hypothalamus signals for water to be consumed. The body must excrete about 500ml each day as urine, which is enough to carry out the waste products generated by a day's worth of metabolic activities (Debruyne, Pinna & Whitney, 2008). Water is also lost as vapor from the lungs, through fecal matter and evaporation from the skin. The general rule of thumb for water intake is to consume roughly 64 ounces, or 8 glasses, of water per day. Your first urine of the day will probably be darker yellow. If, say, by 3 PM, your urine is still dark yellow, then you are probably mildly dehydrated. Mild dehydration can cause headaches, lethargy, rapid pulse, and decreased athletic performance.

It is best to consume fluids through plain old tap or bottled water, but you can also get fluids from milk, soups, and watery fruits.

RESOURCES

American Heart Association: *www.americanheart.org*

Atkins, R. 1999. *Dr. Atkins' New Diet Revolution*. Harper Collins: New York.

Burke, L., Deakin, V. 2000. *Clinical Sports Nutrition*, Roseville, Australia: McGraw-Hill.

Center for Science in the Public Interest (CSPI) 1999. America: Drowning in sugar. *http://www.cspinet.org/new/sugar.html*

DeBruyne, L. K., Pinna, K., Whitney, E. 2008. *Nutrition and Diet Therapy*, 7th ed., Thomson/Wadsworth.

De Oliveira e Silva, E. R. et al. 2000. Alcohol Consumption Raises HDL Cholesterol Levels by Increasing the Transport Rate of Apolipoproteins A-I and A-II. *Circulation*: (102):2347–52.

Dietary Reference Intakes for Energy, Carbohydrate, Fiber, Fat, Fatty Acids, Cholesterol, Protein, and Amino Acids. 2005. *Standing Committee on the Scientific Evaluation of Dietary Reference Intakes*, p. 265.

Foster, G. D., Ph.D., Holly R. Wyatt, M.D., James O. Hill, Ph.D., Brian G. McGuckin, Ed.M., Carrie Brill, B.S., B. Selma Mohammed, M.D., Ph.D., Philippe O. Szapary, M.D., Daniel J. Rader, M.D., Joel S. Edman, D.Sc., and Samuel Klein, M.D. 2003. A Randomized Trial of a Low-Carbohydrate Diet for Obesity. *The New England Journal of Medicine*: Volume (348): 2082–90.

Mahoney, S., Schocker, L. 2010. Should you kick the multivitamin habit? *Prevention*, November, 52–59.

Marlett, J. A., McBurney, M. I., Slavin, J. L. 2002. *Position of the American Dietetic Association: Health Implications of Dietary Fiber* 102, (7):993–1000.

Tipton, K. D. 2004. Ingestion of casein and whey proteins result in muscle anabolism after resistance exercise. *Medicine and Science in Sports and Exercise* (36):33–38.

chapter 4
Diet and Health

Leading causes of death, which include heart disease, high blood pressure, many cancers, diabete,s and stroke, are largely preventable through lifestyle choices. Simple lifestyle changes can save lives and improve a person's quality of life.

Diet related diseases are linked to what we eat and kill an estimated three out of four Americans each year. These diseases include heart disease, high blood pressure, stroke, some types of cancer, and diabetes. Everyone has some degree of risk for developing diet-related chronic diseases, and this risk increases with lifestyle. Lifestyle factors that contribute to increased risk for these diseases include not eating enough fruits and vegetables, eating too many foods high in saturated fats (fried foods, full-fat dairy products, fatty cuts of meat), and not getting enough exercise.

Most Americans don't eat enough fruits and vegetables to keep them healthy. Eating a diet that contains five to nine servings of fruits and vegetables a day as part of a healthy, active lifestyle lowers the risk for all of these diseases. Calories and body weight go hand in hand with developing diet-related diseases. Excess body fat leads to an increased risk of health problems and diet-related diseases that are easily prevented through proper food intake. The earlier a person starts to eat a healthy and balanced diet, the more likely he or she will stay healthy.

The foods we eat contain a variety of vitamins, minerals, and other important nutrients that help keep our bodies healthy. All of these nutrients are needed in balanced proportion. The body cannot function properly if one or more nutrients are missing. A healthy and balanced diet provides foods in the right amounts and combinations that are safe and free from disease and harmful substances.

Food is essential for our bodies to:
- develop, replace, and repair cells and tissues;
- produce energy to keep warm, move, and work;
- carry out chemical processes such as the digestion of food; and
- protect against, resist, and fight infection, and recover from sickness.

Heart disease, which is largely influenced by what we eat, remains the number one killer of both American men and women. High blood pressure, which can be reduced within a month by changing eating habits, will affect 90 percent of American men and women at some point in their lifetime. In general, men get chronic diseases more often than women and die from them at earlier ages. African American men have even higher rates of these diseases than white men, including heart disease, high blood pressure, many cancers, and diabetes, and get them even earlier in life.

HEART DISEASE

Heart disease is a number of abnormal conditions affecting the heart and the blood vessels in the heart. Both men and women have heart attacks, but more women who have heart attacks die from them. One in three American women dies of heart disease. African American and Hispanic American/Latina women are more likely than white women to get heart disease because they tend to have more risk factors such as obesity, lack of exercise, high blood pressure, and diabetes.

Types of heart disease include:

- **Coronary artery disease (CAD)** is the most common type and is the leading cause of heart attacks. Arteries become hard and narrow. Blood has a hard time getting to the heart, so the heart does not get all the blood it needs. CAD can lead to:
  - **Angina.** Angina is chest pain or discomfort that happens when the heart does not get enough blood.
  - **Heart attack.** A heart attack occurs when an artery is severely or completely blocked, and the heart does not get the blood it needs for more than 20 minutes.
- **Heart failure** occurs when the heart is not able to pump blood through the body as well as it should. This means that other organs, which normally get blood from the heart, do not get enough blood.

Symptoms of a heart attack include:

- Pain or discomfort in the center of the chest
- Pain or discomfort in other areas of the upper body, including the arms, back, neck, jaw, or stomach
- Other symptoms, such as shortness of breath (feeling like you can't get enough air), breaking out in a cold sweat, nausea (feeling sick to your stomach), or feeling faint or woozy

Not everyone has all of the warning signs of a heart attack. And, sometimes these signs can go away and come back.

Some women have more vague symptoms such as:

- Unusual tiredness
- Trouble sleeping
- Problems breathing
- Indigestion (upset stomach)
- Anxiety (feeling uneasy or worried)

Suggestions for reducing heart disease risk:

- **Know your blood pressure.** Your heart moves blood through your body. If it is hard for your heart to do this, your heart works harder, and your blood pressure will rise.
- **Do not smoke.** Smoking clogs your arteries.
- **Get tested for diabetes.**
- **Get your cholesterol and triglyceride levels tested.** High blood cholesterol can clog your arteries and keep your heart from getting the blood it needs. This can cause a heart attack. Triglycerides are a form of fat in your blood stream.
- **Maintain a healthy weight.** Being overweight raises your risk for heart disease.

- **Limit alcohol.** If you drink alcohol, limit it to no more than one drink (one 12-ounce beer, one 5-ounce glass of wine, or one 1.5-ounce shot of hard liquor) a day.
- **Cope with stress.** Stress hormones, such as cortisol, increase abdominal obesity and risk of heart disease.

Saturated Fat, Cholesterol, and Heart Disease

Dietary suggestions:

A diet high in saturated fat causes cholesterol, which is a soft, waxy substance, to build up in the arteries. Eventually the arteries harden and narrow. The result is an increased pressure in the arteries and a strain on the heart to maintain adequate blood flow throughout the body, which can cause a heart attack.

There are two types of cholesterol:

- **Low-density lipoprotein** (LDL) is often called the "bad" type of cholesterol because it can clog the arteries that carry blood to your heart.
- **High-density lipoprotein** (HDL) is known as "good" cholesterol because it takes the bad cholesterol out of your blood and keeps it from building up in your arteries.

- **Total cholesterol level**—Lower is better. Less than 200 mg/dL is best.

Total Cholesterol Level	Category
Less than 200 mg/dL	Desirable
200 to 239 mg/dL	Borderline high
240 mg/dL and above	High

- **LDL (bad) cholesterol**—Lower is better. Less than 100 mg/dL is best.

LDL Cholesterol Level	Category
Less than 100 mg/dL	Optimal
100–129 mg/dL	Near optimal/above optimal
130–159 mg/dL	Borderline high
160–189 mg/dL	High
190 mg/dL and above	Very high

- **HDL (good) cholesterol**—Higher is better. More than 60 mg/dL is best.
- **Triglyceride levels**—Lower is better. Less than 150 mg/dL is best.

Eat foods low in saturated fats, trans fats, and cholesterol.

Eat more:

- Fish, poultry (chicken, turkey—breast meat or drumstick is best), and lean meats (round, sirloin, loin). Broil, bake, roast, or poach foods. Remove the fat and skin before eating
- Skim (fat-free) or low-fat (1%) milk and cheeses, and low-fat or nonfat yogurt
- Fruits and vegetables (5 to 9 a day)
- Cereals, breads, rice, and pasta made from whole grains (such as "whole-wheat" or "whole-grain" bread and pasta, rye bread, brown rice, and oatmeal)

Eat less:
- Organ meats (liver, kidney, brains)
- Egg yolks
- Fats (butter, lard) and oils
- Packaged and processed foods

Move more: Exercise can help lower LDL and raise HDL. Exercise at a moderate intensity for at least 30 minutes most days of the week.

Omega-3 Lowers Triglycerides and CVD Risk

Since the first AHA Science Advisory "Fish Consumption, Fish Oil, Lipids, and Coronary Heart Disease," important new findings have been reported about the beneficial effects of omega-3 fatty acids on cardiovascular disease (CVD) in patients with preexisting CVD as well as in healthy individuals. We need omega-3 fatty acids for numerous normal body functions, such as controlling blood clotting and building cell membranes in the brain, and since our bodies cannot make omega-3 fats, we must get them through food. Omega-3 fatty acids are also associated with many health benefits, including protection against heart disease and possibly stroke. New studies are identifying potential benefits for a wide range of conditions including cancer, inflammatory bowel disease, and other autoimmune diseases such as lupus and rheumatoid arthritis.

Triglycerides are a form of fat that is found in your blood. They get in your blood from what you eat. They are found in foods that are high in fat and in particular saturated fat and high sugar foods. Triglycerides can lead to blood clots and they can also cause your HDL (good cholesterol) to lower, which in turn can cause heart disease.

Types of Omega-3 Fatty Acids

The first type is **alpha-linolenic acid (ALA)** and comes from vegetative sources. It is found in . . .

- flaxseed oil
- soybean oil
- canola oil

Less potent sources are . . .

- walnuts
- dairy products
- beans
- broccoli
- green leafy vegetables

The second type of omega-3 comes from the ocean. It includes **eicosapentaenoic acid (EPA)** and **docosahexaenoic acid (DHA).** Both are derived from cold-water fatty fish. Some potent sources are . . .

- salmon
- mackerel
- lake trout
- herring
- sardines
- albacore tuna

Omega-6 fatty acids are also polyunsaturated fatty acids that are essential nutrients, meaning that our bodies cannot make them and we must obtain them from food. Omega-6 fatty acids lower LDL cholesterol (the "bad" cholesterol) and reduce inflammation. They are abundant in the Western diet; common sources include:

- safflower, corn, cottonseed, and soybean oils.

Vitamin D and Prevention of Diseases

Greater Resistance to Viruses

Researchers at the Yale University School of Medicine discovered that people with high levels of vitamin D got sick about half as often as people with low levels. And when they did fall sick, they recovered in fewer days. The reason: Vitamin D instructs your white blood cells to manufacture a protein that kills infections.

Less Cancer and Higher Cancer Survival Rate

Vitamin D has been shown to shut down any out-of-control growth to prevent malignancy as well as helping to kill the cancer cell. And if a tumor grows anyway, it will work to cut off blood supply.

Reduced Risk of Parkinson's

Researchers believe that this is due to vitamin D's protective effect on the brain: It regulates calcium levels, enhances the conduction of electricity through neurons, and detoxifies cells.

Reduced Risk of Heart Disease

People with low vitamin D levels have an 80 percent greater risk of narrowing of the arteries. Researchers say this is due to vitamins D's role in regulating more than 200 genes, controlling inflammation, and in regulating blood pressure.

Diabetes

Vitamin D stimulates insulin production. Research has shown that too little D can cause diabetes and in children deficient in D, a 200 percent greater chance of developing type 1 diabetes has been seen.

Chronic Pain

A 2008 study showed that more than 25 percent of chronic pain patients have low D levels, which could be because D helps control neuromuscular function. And a 2010 study correlated low levels of the vitamin with migraines and headaches.

Depression

Vitamin D may increase serotonin production, which makes you feel calm and happy. Therefore low levels have been linked to depression.

Where Is Vitamin D Found and How Much Is Enough?

Food sources such as fatty fish, eggs, fortified milk, and cod liver oil. As little as 10 minutes of sun is thought to be enough to prevent deficiencies. Adults need 600 IU and children need 400 IU.

Fiber and Coronary Heart Disease

The average American eats 12 grams of fiber a day; most health organizations recommend 20 to 35 grams. Studies have shown that dietary fiber clearly lower blood cholesterol. High-fiber foods are digested more slowly, so they don't cause spikes in blood-sugar levels like white bread, potatoes, and sweets do.

Some fiber, especially soluble fiber, binds to lipids such as cholesterol. The fiber then carries the lipids out of the body through the stool. This lowers the concentration of lipids in the blood and may reduce the risk of coronary heart disease.

Dietary fiber is found in plant foods, where it occurs in two forms: soluble and insoluble. Soluble fiber attracts water and turns to gel during digestion. This process slows digestion and the rate of nutrient absorption from the stomach and intestine. Soluble fiber is found in oat bran, barley, nuts, seeds, dried beans and legumes, lentils, peas, and some fruits and vegetables.

Insoluble fiber also adds bulk (fiber) to the stool. It is found in wheat bran, vegetables, and whole grains.

Soy and Lower Cholesterol

Soy has been shown to significantly lower cholesterol. The right diet can lower cholesterol as much as medication, according to a study reported July 2003 in *The Journal of the American Medical Association.* The four-week study found that a diet of soy fiber, protein from oats and barley, almonds, and margarine from plant sterols lowered cholesterol as much as statins, the most widely prescribed cholesterol medicine. Soybeans themselves provide high-quality protein, are low in saturated fat, and contain no cholesterol, making them an ideal heart-healthy food. To lower your cholesterol, the American Heart Association suggests that you look for products that provide 10 grams of soy protein per serving, and try to eat three or more servings per day (JAMA 2003).

Antioxidants

The carotenoids and anthocyanins that provide the color for fruits and vegetables contain health-enhancing nutrients that protect against heart disease and cancer, and also improve our sense of balance, our memory, and other cognitive skills.

A Handy Guide to Antioxidants

Beta-Carotene

Found in: Orange and yellow fruits and vegetables, such as carrots and cantaloupe; dark leafy greens, such as spinach and kale.

Benefits: Beta-carotene was long believed to help prevent cataracts, although today the research appears to be more conflicted, and scientists say more research is needed.

Lutein

Found in: Leafy greens, such as spinach, corn, carrots, and squash.

Benefits: Research indicates that lutein may help lower the risk of developing cataracts and macular degeneration.

Lycopene

Found in: Red, fleshy fruits and vegetables, such as watermelon and tomatoes.

Benefits: Diets rich in lycopene may help protect against heart disease.

Selenium

Found in: Seafood, lean meats, and whole grains.

Benefits: Research often suggests that selenium may have a preventive effect against cancer.

Vitamin A

Found in: Animal sources such as eggs, meat, and dairy.

Benefits: Research indicates that vitamin A promotes clear and healthy vision. It also helps form and maintain healthy teeth, skeletal and soft tissue, and skin.

Vitamin C

Found in: Citrus fruits, such as oranges and grapefruit; bell peppers; broccoli.

Benefits: Among its many functions, vitamin C can aid tissue growth and repair, adrenal gland function, and wound repair. It may also help cure or prevent colds by boosting the immune system.

Vitamin E

Found in: Wheat germ, nuts (e.g., almonds, walnuts, hazelnuts), and monounsaturated oils (e.g., sunflower oil).

Benefits: Vitamin E acts as a powerful antioxidant by neutralizing free radicals in the body that cause tissue and cellular damage. Vitamin E also contributes to a healthy circulatory system and aids in proper blood clotting and improves wound healing.

American Heart Association Dietary Recommendations

- Vegetables and fruits are high in vitamins, minerals, and fiber, and low in calories. Eating a variety of fruits and vegetables may help you control your weight and your blood pressure.
- Unrefined whole-grain foods contain fiber that can help lower your blood cholesterol and help you feel full, which may help you manage your weight.
- Eat fish at least twice a week. Recent research shows that eating oily fish containing omega-3 fatty acids (for example, salmon, trout, and herring) may help lower your risk of death from coronary artery disease.
- Choose lean meats and poultry without skin and prepare them without added saturated and trans fat.
- Select fat-free, 1% fat, and low-fat dairy products.
- Cut back on foods containing partially hydrogenated vegetable oils to reduce *trans* fat in your diet.
- Cut back on foods high in dietary cholesterol. Aim to eat less than 300 milligrams of cholesterol each day.
- Cut back on beverages and foods with added sugars.

- Choose and prepare foods with little or no salt. Aim to eat less than 2,300 milligrams of sodium per day.
- If you drink alcohol, drink in moderation, which means one drink per day if you're a woman and two drinks per day if you're a man.

HYPERTENSION (HIGH BLOOD PRESSURE)

Hypertension (high blood pressure) affects one in four adults in the United States. High blood pressure is often called the "silent killer" because it has no symptoms and can go undetected for years. Your blood pressure is the force exerted on your artery walls by the blood flowing through your body. A blood pressure reading provides two measures, systolic pressure and diastolic pressure, which are expressed as millimeters of mercury (mm Hg), or how high the pressure of blood would raise a column of mercury. Systolic pressure is measured as the heart pumps. Diastolic pressure is measured between beats, as blood flows back into the heart.

Hypertension cannot be cured, but it can be controlled through lifestyle changes and prescriptive medication. Although medications to treat hypertension are available, research has shown that modest lifestyle and dietary changes can help treat and often delay or prevent high blood pressure. Untreated hypertension causes damage to the blood vessels over time, which can lead to other health complications, such as strokes, kidney failure, impaired vision, heart attack, and heart failure.

Know Your Numbers

	Systolic (MM HG)		Diastolic (MM HG)
Normal	<120	and	<80
Prehypertension	120–139	or	80–89
HYPERTENSION			
Stage 1	140–159	or	90–99
Stage 2	≥160	or	≤100

Dietary Recommendations:

Salt isn't the only source of sodium in our food. When you're reading food labels, be on the lookout for:

- sodium
- rock salt
- monosodium glutamate (MSG)
- sea salt
- Sodium alginate
- Sodium ascorbate
- Sodium bicarbonate (baking soda)
- Sodium benzoate
- Sodium caseinate
- Sodium chloride
- Sodium citrate

- Sodium hydroxide
- Sodium saccharin
- Monosodium glutamate

People trying to control hypertension often are advised to decrease sodium, increase potassium, watch their calories, and maintain a reasonable weight.

- The recommendation for daily sodium intake is 1,500 to 2,300 mg a day. Table salt is 40 percent sodium. One teaspoon has about 2,000 mg sodium.
- Potassium works with sodium to regulate the body's water balance. Research has shown that the more potassium and less sodium a person has in his or her diet, the greater the likelihood that the person will maintain normal blood pressure. However, the evidence does not suggest that people with high blood pressure should take potassium supplements. Instead, potassium rich foods should be eaten every day.
- People with a low calcium intake seem to be at increased risk for hypertension. Everyone should meet the dietary reference intake (DRI) for calcium every day.
- For people who are overweight, even a small weight loss can dramatically reduce or even prevent high blood pressure.
- Incorporate the DASH diet into your lifestyle. A landmark study called DASH (Dietary Approaches to Stop Hypertension) looked at the effects of an overall eating plan in adults with normal to high blood pressure. Researchers found that in just eight weeks, people following the DASH diet saw their blood pressure decrease. A subsequent study called DASH 2 looked at the effect of following the DASH diet and restricting salt intake to 1,500 mg per day. Under the DASH 2 diet, people with Stage 1 hypertension had their blood pressure decrease as much or more than any anti-hypertensive medication had been able to lower it.

Strategies for Meeting the DASH diet:

- Eat more fruits, vegetables, and low-fat dairy foods.
- Cut back on foods that are high in saturated fat, cholesterol, and total fat.
- Eat more whole grain products, fish, poultry, and nuts.
- Eat less red meat and sweets.
- Eat foods that are rich in magnesium, potassium, and calcium.

The DASH Diet

Food Group	Daily Servings	Significance to the DASH Diet
Grains and grain products	7 to 8	Carbohydrates and fiber
Vegetables	4 to 5	Potassium, magnesium, and fiber
Fruits	4 to 5	Potassium, magnesium, and fiber
Low-fat or fat-free milk or milk products	2 to 3	Calcium, protein, potassium, and magnesium
Meats, poultry, and fish	2 or less	Protein and magnesium
Nuts, seeds, and beans	4 to 5 a week	Magnesium, potassium, protein, and fiber

DIABETES

Diabetes is the sixth leading cause of death in the United States. About 65 percent of deaths among those with diabetes are attributed to heart disease and stroke. The disease often leads to blindness, heart and blood vessel disease, stroke, kidney failure, amputations, and nerve damage. Uncontrolled diabetes can complicate pregnancy, and birth defects are more common in babies born to women with diabetes.

According to recent estimates from the Centers for Disease Control and Prevention (CDC), diabetes will affect one in three people born in 2000 in the United States. The CDC also projects the prevalence of diagnosed diabetes in the United States will increase 165 percent by 2050. Diabetes prevalence in the United States is likely to increase for several reasons. First, a large segment of the population is aging. Also, Hispanics/Latinos and other minority groups at increased risk make up the fastest-growing segment of the U.S. population. Finally, Americans are increasingly overweight and sedentary. Source: *http://www.cdc.gov/nccdphp/publications/aag/ddt.htm*

Diabetes is a disorder of metabolism, the way our bodies use digested food for growth and energy. Most of the food we eat is broken down into glucose, the form of sugar in the blood. Glucose is the main source of fuel for the body. After digestion, glucose passes into the bloodstream, where it is used by cells for growth and energy. For glucose to get into cells, insulin must be present. Insulin is a hormone produced by the pancreas, a large gland behind the stomach. When we eat, the pancreas automatically produces the right amount of insulin to move glucose from blood into our cells. In people with diabetes, however, the pancreas either produces little or no insulin, or the cells do not respond appropriately to the insulin that is produced. Glucose builds up in the blood, overflows into the urine, and passes out of the body in the urine. Thus, the body loses its main source of fuel even though the blood contains large amounts of glucose.

How is diabetes diagnosed?

The fasting blood glucose test is the preferred test for diagnosing diabetes in children and non-pregnant adults. It is most reliable when done in the morning.

- A blood glucose level of 126 milligrams per deciliter (mg/dL) or more after an 8-hour fast. This test is called the fasting blood glucose test.
- A blood glucose level of 200 mg/dL or more 2 hours after drinking a beverage containing 75 grams of glucose dissolved in water. This test is called the oral glucose tolerance test (OGTT).
- A random (taken at any time of day) blood glucose level of 200 mg/dL or more, along with the presence of diabetes symptoms.

The three main types of diabetes are:

- Type 1 diabetes
- Type 2 diabetes
- Gestational diabetes

Type 1 Diabetes

Type 1 diabetes is an autoimmune disease. An autoimmune disease results when the body's system for fighting infection (the immune system) turns against a part of the body. In diabetes, the immune system attacks and destroys the insulin-producing beta cells in the pancreas. The pancreas then produces little or no insulin. A person who has type 1 diabetes must take insulin daily to live.

At present, scientists do not know exactly what causes the body's immune system to attack the beta cells, but they believe that autoimmune, genetic, and environmental factors, possibly viruses, are involved. Type 1 diabetes accounts for about 5 to 10 percent of diagnosed diabetes in the United States. It develops most often in children and young adults but it can appear at any age. If not diagnosed and treated with insulin, a person with type 1 diabetes can lapse into a life-threatening diabetic coma, also known as diabetic ketoacidosis.

Symptoms may include:

- Increased thirst and urination
- Constant hunger
- Weight loss
- Blurred vision
- Extreme fatigue

Type 2 Diabetes

The most common form of diabetes is type 2 diabetes. About 90 to 95 percent of people with diabetes have type 2. About 80 percent of people with type 2 diabetes are overweight.

In type 2 diabetes, the pancreas is usually producing enough insulin, but for unknown reasons the body cannot use the insulin effectively, a condition called insulin resistance. After several years, insulin production decreases. The result is the same as for type 1 diabetes; glucose builds up in the blood and the body cannot make efficient use of its main source of fuel.

Symptoms may include:

- Fatigue
- Frequent urination
- Increased thirst and hunger
- Weight loss
- Blurred vision
- Slow healing of wounds or sores

Gestational Diabetes

Some women develop gestational diabetes late in pregnancy. Although this form of diabetes usually disappears after the birth of the baby, women who have had gestational diabetes have a 20 to 50 percent chance of developing type 2 diabetes within 5 to 10 years. Maintaining a reasonable body weight and being physically active may help prevent development of type 2 diabetes.

Gestational diabetes is caused by the hormones of pregnancy or a shortage of insulin. Women with gestational diabetes may not experience any symptoms.

Nutrition Suggestions:

Healthful eating helps keep your blood glucose, also called blood sugar, in your target range. Physical activity and, if needed, diabetes medicines also help.

The diabetes food pyramid divides foods into groups, based on what they contain. A person with diabetes must eat more from the groups at the bottom of the pyramid, and less from the groups at the top. Foods from the starches, fruits, vegetables, and milk groups are highest in carbohydrate. They affect blood glucose levels the most.

Target Blood Glucose Levels for People with Diabetes

Before meals	70 to 130
1 to 2 hours after the start of a meal	less than 180

The Diabetes Food Pyramid

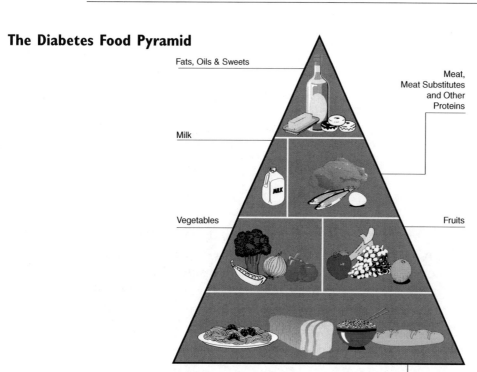

Source: Adapted from *http://diabetes.niddk.nih.gov/*

Have about 1,200 to 1,600 calories a day if you are a:

- small woman who exercises
- small or medium-sized woman who wants to lose weight
- medium-sized woman who does not exercise much

Choose this many servings from these food groups to have **1,200 to 1,600 calories** a day:	
6 starches	2 milks
3 vegetables	4 to 6 ounces meat and meat substitutes
2 fruits	up to 3 fats

Have about 1,600 to 2,000 calories a day if you are a:

- large woman who wants to lose weight
- small man at a healthy weight
- medium-sized man who does not exercise much
- medium-sized or large man who wants to lose weight

Choose this many servings from these food groups to have **1,600 to 2,000 calories** a day:	
8 starches	2 milks
4 vegetables	4 to 6 ounces meat and meat substitutes
3 fruits	up to 4 fats

Have about 2,000 to 2,400 calories a day if you are a:

- medium-sized or large man who exercises a lot or has a physically active job
- large man at a healthy weight
- medium-sized or large woman who exercises a lot or has a physically active job

Choose this many servings from these food groups to have **2,000 to 2,400 calories** a day:	
10 starches	2 milks
4 vegetables	5 to 7 ounces meat and meat substitutes
4 fruits	up to 5 fats

Osteoporosis

Osteoporosis is a major public health threat for 44 million Americans—68 percent of whom are women. Osteoporosis is a disease characterized by low bone mass and structural deterioration of bone tissue, leading to bone fragility and an increased risk of fractures. Osteoporosis is a disease in which the calcium content of bones is very low. In this disease, calcium and phosphorus, which are normally present in the bones, become reabsorbed back into the body. This process results in brittle, fragile bones that are easily broken.

Throughout your lifetime, old bone is removed (resorption) and new bone is added to the skeleton (formation). During childhood and teenage years, new bone is added faster than old bone is removed. As a result, bones become larger, heavier, and denser. Bone formation outpaces resorption until peak bone mass (maximum bone density and strength) is reached around age 30.

Risk factors you cannot change:

- *Gender*—Your chances of developing osteoporosis are greater if you are a woman. Women have less bone tissue and lose bone faster than men because of the changes that happen with menopause.
- *Age*—The older you are, the greater your risk of osteoporosis. Your bones become thinner and weaker as you age.
- *Body size*—Small, thin-boned women are at greater risk.
- *Ethnicity*—Caucasian and Asian women are at highest risk. African American and Hispanic women have a lower but significant risk.
- *Family history*—Fracture risk may be due, in part, to heredity. People whose parents have a history of fractures also seem to have reduced bone mass and may be at risk for fractures.

Risk factors you can change:

- *Sex hormones*—Abnormal absence of menstrual periods (amenorrhea), low estrogen level (menopause), and low testosterone level in men can bring on osteoporosis.
- *Anorexia nervosa*—Characterized by an irrational fear of weight gain, this eating disorder increases your risk for osteoporosis.
- *Calcium and vitamin D intake*—A lifetime diet low in calcium and vitamin D makes you more prone to bone loss.
- *Medication use*—Long-term use of glucocorticoids and some anticonvulsants can lead to loss of bone density and fractures.
- *Lifestyle*—An inactive lifestyle or extended bed rest tends to weaken bones.
- *Cigarette smoking*—Cigarettes are bad for bones, as well as the heart and lungs.
- *Alcohol intake*—Excessive consumption increases the risk of bone loss and fractures.

Calcium and Osteoporosis

Dietary suggestions:

The body uses calcium to form and maintain healthy bones and teeth. Calcium also plays a vital role in nerve conduction, muscle contraction, and blood clotting. Getting enough calcium in the diet throughout childhood and puberty is one way to prevent osteoporosis.

The body's demand for calcium is greater during childhood and adolescence, when the skeleton is growing rapidly, and during pregnancy and breastfeeding. Postmenopausal women and older men also need to consume more calcium. Also, as you age, your body becomes less efficient at absorbing calcium and other nutrients. Older adults also are more likely to have chronic medical problems and to use medications that may impair calcium absorption. Add calcium-rich foods such as low-fat cheese and milk to your diet. Researchers at Purdue University found that people who consume calcium from low-fat dairy products, or get at least 1,000 milligrams a day, showed an overall decrease in body weight.

- Choose skim milk, low-fat yogurt, and low-fat cheese to avoid saturated fats. A single serving can provide you with 20 percent of the 1,200 milligrams a day you need.
- Add calcium-enriched cereals, breads, and orange juice to your diet.
- Consume foods that are dark green, leafy vegetables, such as broccoli, collard greens, bok choy, and spinach; sardines and salmon with bones; tofu; and almonds.
- Consider taking a calcium supplement.
- Add weight-bearing exercise. Like muscle, bone is living tissue that responds to exercise by becoming stronger. Weight-bearing exercise is the best for your bones because it forces you to work against gravity. Examples include walking, hiking, jogging, stair climbing, weight training, tennis, and dancing.
- Vitamin D plays an important role in calcium absorption and in bone health. It is made in the skin through exposure to sunlight. Depending on your situation, you may need to take vitamin D supplements to ensure a daily intake of between 400 to 800 IU of vitamin D.
- Give up smoking. Smoking is bad for your bones. Smokers also may absorb less calcium from their diets.
- Alcohol: Regular consumption of 2 to 3 ounces a day of alcohol may be damaging to the skeleton, even in young women and men. Those who drink heavily are more prone to bone loss and fractures, because of both poor nutrition and increased risk of falling.

Recommended Calcium Intakes (mg/day)
National Academy of Sciences

Ages	mg/day
Birth–6 months	210
6 months–1 year	270
1–3	500
4–8	800
9–13	1300
14–18	1300
19–30	1000
31–50	1000
51–70	1200
70 or older	1200
Pregnant or lactating	
14–18	1300
19–50	1000

NUTRITION FOR THE CANCER PATIENT

Half of all men and one-third of all women in the United States will develop cancer during their lifetimes. The risk of developing most types of cancer can be reduced by changes in a person's lifestyle, for example, by quitting smoking, limiting time in the sun, being physically active, and eating a better diet.

Cancer is the general name for a group of more than 100 diseases in which cells in a part of the body begin to grow out of control. Normal body cells grow, divide, and die in an orderly fashion. Cancer cells develop because of damage to DNA, which is a substance in every cell and directs all of the cell's activities. Most of the time when DNA becomes damaged, either the cell dies or is able to repair the DNA. In cancer cells, the damaged DNA is not repaired. People can inherit damaged DNA, which accounts for inherited cancers. Many times though, a person's DNA gets damaged by things in the environment, like chemicals, viruses, tobacco smoke, too much sunlight, or improper nutrition.

Because cancer cells keep growing and dividing, they are different from normal cells. Instead of dying, they outlive normal cells and continue to grow and make new, abnormal cells. Cancer usually forms as a tumor (a lump or mass.) Some cancers, like leukemia, do not form tumors; instead, these cancer cells involve the blood and blood-forming organs, and circulate through other tissues where they grow. Cancer cells often travel through the bloodstream or through the lymph system to other parts of the body where they begin to grow and replace normal tissue. This spreading process is called metastasis. Benign (non-cancerous) tumors do not spread to other parts of the body (metastasize) and are very rarely life-threatening.

Fiber and Cancer

Studies have shown that a diet high in nutrients and fiber can reduce the risk of developing cancers of the stomach, colon, rectum, esophagus, larynx, and lung.

Fruits, Vegetables, and Cancer

Eating more fruits and vegetables helps provide a good supply of fiber, vitamin A, vitamin C, beta carotene and other carotenoids, and phytochemicals which are plant chemicals that may affect human health. There are hundreds of phytochemicals, and their exact role in promoting health is still unclear. However, a growing body of evidence indicates that phytochemicals may help protect against cancer.

Vitamin C and beta carotene, which forms vitamin A, are antioxidants. They protect body cells from oxidation, a process that can lead to cell damage and may play a role in cancer. Antioxidants include dark-green, leafy vegetables such as spinach, kale, collards, and turnip greens. Citrus fruits, such as oranges, grapefruit, and tangerines are also high in antioxidants. Other red, yellow, and orange fruits and vegetables—or their juices—are also healthful choices.

Alcohol and Cancer

Alcohol is processed by the liver into energy for the body. Continued and excessive use of alcohol can damage the liver in various ways, including the development of a fatty liver. A fatty liver can lead to cirrhosis of the liver. Alcohol use also increases the risk of liver cancer. When combined with smoking, alcohol intake also increases the risk of cancers of the mouth, throat, larynx, and esophagus. In addition, alcohol intake is associated with an increased risk of breast cancer in women.

Alcohol can damage the lining of the small intestine and stomach, where most nutrients are digested. As a result, alcohol can impair the absorption of essential nutrients. Alcohol also increases the body's need for some nutrients, and interferes with the absorption and storage of other nutrients.

If you choose to drink alcohol, do so in moderation. Limit yourself to no more than 2 drinks per day if male, 1 per day if female.

Nitrates and Cancer

Countries in which people eat a lot of salt-cured, smoked, and nitrite-cured foods have a high rate of cancer of the stomach and esophagus. Examples of such foods include bacon, ham, hot dogs, and salt-cured fish.

Fat and Cancer

A diet high in fat has been shown to increase the risk of cancers of the breast, colon, and prostate. A diet high in fat may promote cancer by causing the body to secrete more of certain hormones that create a favorable environment for certain types of cancer. High-fat diets also may change the characteristics of the cells to make them more vulnerable to cancer-causing agents.

To reduce fat in the diet, choose lean cuts of beef, lamb, and pork, as well as skinless poultry and fish. Baking, broiling, poaching, and steaming are recommended cooking methods. Choose skim or low-fat milk and dairy products, as well as low-fat salad dressings.

Nutrition Suggestions for People Getting Radiation Therapy

In radiation therapy, radiation is directed at the parts of the body with cancer so the cells are unable to grow and divide. People with cancer often get radiation treatments 5 days a week for 2 to 9 weeks.

The type of side effects that radiation may cause depends on the area of the body being treated, the size of the area being treated, the total dose of radiation, and the number of treatments.

Some common side effects include:
- Nausea
- Hair loss
- Fatigue
- Low blood count
- Inflammation inside the mouth
- Sensitive skin

Dietary suggestions:
- Try to eat something at least 60 minutes before treatment rather than going in with an empty stomach.
- Salty foods or ice cold drinks help control nausea.
- Avoid greasy, strong-smelling, or overly sweet foods.
- Drink plenty of water and other liquids.
- Try to eat small, frequent meals and snacks rather than three large meals and eat them slowly. If your appetite is better at certain times of the day, plan on having your largest meal then.
- Nutrition supplements, such as liquid meal replacements, can be helpful during this time.

Nutrition Suggestions for People Getting Chemotherapy

Chemotherapy involves taking strong drugs that kill cancer cells. The drugs are most commonly taken by mouth or given by injection into the bloodstream. Chemotherapy drugs can damage both healthy cells and cancer cells.

Common side effects of chemotherapy that can cause eating problems:
- Loss of appetite
- Changes in taste and smell
- Mouth tenderness or sores
- Nausea
- Vomiting
- Changes in bowel habits
- Fatigue
- Low white blood cell counts with the increased risk of infection

Dietary suggestions:
- Eat something before getting treatment.
- Eat a balanced diet that includes protein (meat, milk, eggs, and beans, lentils, and other legumes) to help boost your energy. (Chemotherapy patients are often very tired.)
- Eat small, frequent meals or snacks.
- Go easy on fried or greasy foods. These can be hard to digest.
- Drink plenty of water or liquids (eight to ten 8-oz glasses) each day.

HIV/AIDS AND NUTRITION

Good nutrition is vital to help maintain the health and quality of life of the person suffering from HIV/AIDS. When nutritional needs are not met, recovery from an illness will take longer. The HIV virus attacks the immune system. In the early stages of infection, a person shows no visible signs of illness, but later many of the signs of AIDS will become apparent, including weight loss, fever, diarrhea, and opportunistic infections (such as sore throat and tuberculosis). These infections can lower food intake because they both reduce appetite and interfere with the body's ability to absorb food. As a result, the person becomes malnourished, loses weight, and is weakened.

Food, once eaten, is broken down by digestion into nutrients. These nutrients pass through the gut walls into the bloodstream and are transported to the organs and tissues in the body where they are needed. One of the consequences of HIV, cancer, and other infections is that because the gut wall is damaged, food does not pass through properly and is consequently not absorbed. When a person does not eat enough food, or the food eaten is poorly absorbed, the body draws on its reserve stores of energy from body fat and protein from muscle. As a result, the person loses weight because body weight and muscles are lost. For an average adult, serious weight loss is indicated by a 10 percent loss of body weight or 6 to 7 kg in one month.

People with HIV/AIDS often do not eat enough because:

- the illness and the medicines taken for it may reduce the appetite, modify the taste of food and prevent the body from absorbing it;
- symptoms such as a sore mouth, nausea, and vomiting make it difficult to eat; and
- fatigue, isolation, and depression reduce the appetite and the willingness to make an effort to prepare food and eat regularly.

Suggestions for gaining weight: Weight is gained by eating more food, either by eating larger portions and/or eating meals more frequently, and using a variety of foods.

- Eat more starchy foods such as rice, pasta, wheat, bread, potatoes, sweet potatoes, yams, and bananas.
- Increase intake of beans, soy products, lentils, peas, groundnuts, peanut butter, and seeds, such as sunflower and sesame.
- Include all forms of meat, poultry, fish, and eggs as often as possible.
- Eat snacks regularly between meals. Good snacks are nuts, seeds, fruit, yogurt, and peanut butter sandwiches.
- Slowly increase the fat content of the food by using more fats and oils, as well as avocados.
- Introduce more dairy products.
- Add dry milk powder to foods such as porridge, cereals, sauces, and mashed potatoes.
- Add sugar, honey, jam, and syrup to the food.
- Make meals as attractive as possible.

Increase Exercise

Exercise is especially important for maintaining the health of people with HIV/AIDS. Regular exercise makes a person feel more alert, helps to relieve stress, and stimulates the appetite. Exercise is the only way to strengthen and build up muscles. The body uses muscles to store energy and protein that the immune system can draw upon when required.

GLUTEN INTOLERANCE AND CELIAC DISEASE

People who have celiac disease have a form of autoimmune disease and cannot tolerate gluten, a protein in wheat, rye, and barley. Celiac disease is a digestive disease that damages the villi of the small intestine and interferes with absorption of nutrients from food. Nutrition therapy which eliminates foods with gluten is the only treatment.

Rice, potato or corn flour, buckwheat, soy, tapioca, and quinoa are substituted for wheat, rye, and barley that contain gluten which are in many foods. Oats are only allowed if they are manufactured in a plant not manufacturing or milling any wheat, rye, or barley ingredients. Vegetable protein products such as veggie burgers may contain wheat and soy.

Symptoms

- abdominal bloating and pain
- chronic diarrhea
- vomiting
- constipation
- pale, foul-smelling, or fatty stool
- weight loss
- unexplained iron-deficiency anemia
- fatigue
- bone or joint pain
- arthritis
- bone loss or osteoporosis
- depression or anxiety
- tingling numbness in the hands and feet
- seizures
- missed menstrual periods
- infertility or recurrent miscarriage
- canker sores inside the mouth
- an itchy skin rash

Beware of Dangerous Food and Medication Interactions

Some drugs interfere with the body's ability to absorb nutrients, and some foods can lessen or increase the impact of a drug.

- **Grapefruit and grapefruit juice** can interact in a dangerous way with certain medications. Ex: blood pressure medications such as Procardia and Adalat (Nifedipine) and Plendil (felodipine), will result in higher levels of these blood pressure medications, and side effects include facial flushing, nausea, dizziness, confusion, palpitations, or irregular heartbeat.
- **Green, leafy vegetables,** such as broccoli, brussels sprouts and cabbage can reduce the effectiveness of the blood thinner Coumadin (warfarin), which is a very commonly prescribed blood thinner that is used to prevent blood clots. These foods are rich in vitamin K, which helps the blood to clot, so the interaction can reduce the drug's effectiveness and put one at risk for blood clot or stroke.

- **Oatmeal and other high fiber foods** are believed to interfere with the absorption of Lanoxin (digoxin), a drug that is frequently prescribed to control an irregular heart rhythm.
- **Salt substitutes and diuretics**—contain high amounts of potassium. Salt substitutes are used by people who have high blood pressure. The interaction can make your potassium levels skyrocket, which then may increase your risk of cardiac arrest.
- **Licorice and** diuretics such as Lasix (furosemide) can lead to very low levels of potassium which may lead to an irregular heart rhythm and possibly cardiac arrest.

NUTRITION ASSIGNMENT #4

Case Study

Lisa is a 46-year-old Hispanic female who is 5 feet 6 inches tall and 180 pounds. Lisa has a family history of coronary heart disease and diabetes. Two weeks ago, before her doctor's appointment, a random glucose test performed with a blood glucose meter at a local health fair revealed 180 mg/dl. Her LDL cholesterol was 162 mg/dl and total cholesterol 240 mg/dl. Triglycerides were 300mg/dl. Her blood pressure was 180/100, and fasting blood glucose was 124. She takes diuretics and high blood pressure meds.

Once an avid runner, Lisa has become less physically active in the past year, and her exercise consists of 30 minutes of low-intensity physical activity two times per week. Lisa typically eats 2 cups of frosted flakes cereal, 12 oz. of milk, and grapefruit juice for breakfast. Her lunch consists of one ham sandwich, a Snapple iced tea, and a large fruit salad. Her main meal is a late dinner of large portions of Mexican food (such as enchiladas with rice) or lamb chops with potatoes with milk, and cookies as her late night snack. Her average daily caloric intake is 2,500 kcal/day.

1. What disease(s) is Lisa at risk for and why?

    _____

    _____

    _____

    _____

    _____

    _____

    _____

    _____

    _____

    _____

    _____

    _____

    _____

    _____

    _____

    _____

2. Design a plan of action for Lisa that includes a new diet, caloric expenditure, and exercise reg-
    imen. Should she be aware of any food/drug interactions?

    _____

    _____

    _____

    _____

    _____

    _____

    _____

    _____

    _____

    _____

    _____

    _____

    _____

    _____

    _____

    _____

    _____

RESOURCES

A Clinical Trial of the Effects of Dietary Patterns on Blood Pressure. 1997. *New England Journal of Medicine*, 336:1117–24.

American Cancer Society: *www.cancer.org.*

American Dietetic Association: *www.eatright.org.*

American Heart Association: *www.americanheart.org.*

Centers for Disease Control and Prevention: Diabetes Disabling Disease to Double by 2050: *http://www.cdc.gov/nccdphp/publications/aag/ddt.htm.*

DASHing to Lower Blood Pressure: *www.ext.colostate.edu/PUBS/FOODNUT/09374.html.*

Diet First, Then Medication for Hypercholesterolemia. 2003. *Journal of the American Medical Association*. 290:531–33.

Effects of a Dietary Portfolio of Cholesterol-Lowering Foods vs Lovastatin on Serum Lipids and C-Reactive Protein. 2003. *Journal of the American Medical Association*. 290(4):502–10.

Krauss R. M., Eckel, R. H., Howard, B., et al. AHA Dietary Guidelines: revision 2000: a statement for healthcare professionals from the Nutrition Committee of the American Heart Association. *Circulation*. 2000. 102:2284–99.

The National Cancer Institute's CancerNet: *www.cancer.gov.*

National Cholesterol Education Program, National Heart, Lung, and Blood Institute (NHLBI): *http://www.nhlbi.nih.gov/about/ncep/.*

The National Heart, Lung, and Blood Institute: *www.nhlbi.nih.gov/.*

National High Blood Pressure Education Program, National Heart, Lung, and Blood Institute (NHLBI): http://www.nhlbi.nih.gov/about/nhbpep/index.htm

The National Osteoporosis Foundation: *www.nof.org.*

WomenHeart: *www.womenheart.org.*

chapter 5
Lifecycle Nutrition

In this chapter, you will gain a basic understanding of the nutritional requirements of normal healthy people over the entire lifespan incorporating the special needs of infancy and childhood, adolescence, old age, and pregnancy. You will learn the principles of nutrition assessment for different age groups, gain an understanding of the different nutrient requirements over the life cycle, and learn how the dietary recommendations for nutrient intakes are derived and applied to different populations.

INFANT NUTRITION

Food provides the energy and nutrients a baby or toddler needs to be healthy. Ensuring infants receive adequate nutrients, served in a safe and age-appropriate way, during their first year is essential to their growth and development.

For a baby, breast milk has all the necessary vitamins and minerals. Infant formulas imitate breast milk. Whenever possible, breast milk is best during the first year of life. If breast-feeding isn't possible, an iron-fortified infant formula is an acceptable alternative. Specialized formulas are available if an infant is allergic to regular infant formulas. The baby's pediatrician can advise on the best choice. Proper formula dilution, mixing, and storage are very important. Follow directions carefully. Do not heat baby bottles in the microwave. The Centers for Disease Control and Prevention warn that children's mouths and throats can be severely burned by bottles heated in the microwave.

Nutrition Guidelines
- Children who are younger than 2 years old should obtain up to 50 percent of calories from fat.
- Whole milk is a good source of fat **after age 1.** You can switch to low-fat milk after age 2 or 3. Avoid serving regular cow's milk until infants are 1-year-old. Before then, infants may experience an allergic reaction, stomachache, and low blood iron.
- Ensure that your child gets enough iron.
- Toddlers between 1 and 3 need 500 milligrams of calcium each day.
- Dietary fiber is important after age 3 because it might prevent diseases later on in life.
- Don't feed a baby eggs, citrus fruits and juices, cow's milk, or honey until after his or her first birthday.
- Don't feed the child seafood, peanuts, or tree nuts before age 2 or 3.
- It's important to wash your hands before preparing food or formula for a baby. Not washing hands could result in infant diarrhea from the bacteria picked up by hands in the activities cited.

- Hold the baby when bottle-feeding. Babies who are put to bed with a bottle are more likely to have cavities. There is also a possibility of choking.
- The American Academy of Pediatrics (AAP) recommends giving juice only to infants who are approximately 6 months or older and who can drink from a cup. AAP recommends offering no more than a total of 4 to 6 ounces of juice a day to infants.
- Do not serve infants honey or corn syrup during the first year of life. These foods may contain botulism spores which could cause illness or death in infants.
- AAP recommends breast milk or a prepared iron-fortified infant formula be the only nutrient fed to infants until 4 to 6 months of age.
- When introducing new foods, try only one at a time and start with single-ingredient foods. Avoid serving mixed ingredient foods until each food has been given separately so you can tell if a baby is allergic to a specific food. Begin by serving about 1 to 2 tablespoons and then increase the amount as baby wants more. Wait a week before trying another new food so you can identify any allergic reactions to it.
- Iron-fortified rice cereal is usually the first cereal offered, as babies are least likely to be allergic to it. It's frequently recommended to continue fortified baby cereal through the first year of life.
- Infants may be allergic to egg whites. Wait until about 12 months before offering this food. They may be able to tolerate egg yolks around 8 months.
- Avoid feeding directly from the baby food jar. Bacteria from a baby's mouth can grow and multiply in the food before it is served again. Too many bacteria can make a baby sick. Refrigerate food remaining in the jar and use within 1 to 2 days after opening.
- Do not heat baby foods in their original containers in the microwave. The heat is uneven and can produce "hot spots" that can scald a baby's mouth and throat. Also, the food in the jar may "blow up" in your microwave.
- Once food is opened, don't leave baby food solids or liquids at room temperature for more than 2 hours. Bacteria can grow to harmful levels when food is left out longer than this.
- Avoid serving foods that may choke an infant, such as nuts and seeds, raw carrots and celery, whole kernel corn, raisins, large chunks of meat or cheese, popcorn, chips, pretzels, adult dry cereal, grapes, berries, cherries, unpeeled fruits and vegetables, hard candies, pickles, hot dogs, marshmallows (regular or miniature), and peanut butter. In general, avoid foods that are round and firm, sticky, or cut in large chunks.

TODDLER NUTRITION

Babies grow at a lightning pace 3 inches (8 centimeters) or so every 3 months. A toddler, in contrast, grows at a much slower rate, only 3 to 5 inches (8 to 13 centimeters) in an entire year.

The toddler years are a time of transition, especially between 12 to 24 months, when they're learning to eat table food and accepting new tastes and textures. Depending on their age, size, and activity level, toddlers need about 1,000 to 1,400 calories a day. Fat intake should not be restricted in an infant's diet, but by age 2, a toddler should get only 30 to 35% of daily calories from fat.

Calcium

Children under age 2 should have whole milk to help provide the dietary fats that they need for normal growth and brain development. After age 2, most children can switch to low-fat or nonfat milk. Toddlers should have 500 milligrams of calcium a day. This requirement is easily met if a child gets the recommended two servings of dairy foods every day. An important part of a toddler's diet, milk provides calcium and vitamin D to help build strong bones. Some children don't like milk or are unable to drink or eat dairy products. Explore other calcium sources, such as fortified cereals, calcium-fortified soy beverages, broccoli, and calcium-fortified orange juice.

Drinking a lot of cow's milk (more than 24 to 36 ounces/720 milliliters) also can put a child at risk of developing iron deficiency. Toddlers who drink a lot of cow's milk may be less hungry and less likely to eat iron-rich foods. Milk decreases the absorption of iron and can also irritate the lining of the intestine, causing small amounts of bleeding and the gradual loss of iron in the stool.

Iron

Iron deficiency can affect growth and may lead to learning and behavioral problems and anemia (a decreased number of red blood cells in the body). Iron is needed to make red blood cells, which carry oxygen throughout the body. Without enough iron and red blood cells, the body's tissues and organs get less oxygen and do not function as well.

Toddlers should have 7 milligrams of iron each day. After 12 months of age, toddlers are at risk for iron deficiency because they no longer drink iron-fortified formula and may not be eating iron-fortified infant cereal or enough other iron-containing foods to make up the difference.

To Help Prevent Iron Deficiency:

- Limit a child's milk intake to about 16 to 24 ounces (480 to 720 milliliters) a day.
- Serve more iron-rich foods (meat, poultry, fish, enriched grains, beans, tofu).
- When serving iron-rich meals, include foods that contain vitamin C (tomatoes, broccoli, oranges, and strawberries), which improve the body's iron absorption.
- Continue serving iron-fortified cereal until the child is 18 to 24 months of age.

Nutrition Guidelines for Toddlers

Food Group	Daily Amount for 2-Year-Olds	Daily Amount for 3-Year-Olds	Servings
Grains	3 ounces (85 grams), half from whole-grain sources	4 to 5 ounces (110 to 140 grams), half from whole-grain sources	One ounce equals: 1 slice of bread, 1 cup of ready-to-eat cereal, or ½ cup of cooked rice, cooked pasta, or cooked cereal
Vegetables	1 cup	1.5 cups	Serve vegetables that are soft, cut in small pieces, and well-cooked to prevent choking
Fruits	1 cup	1 to 1½ cups	An 8- to 9-inch (20 to 23 centimeter) banana equals 1 cup
Milk	2 cups (475 milliliters)	2 cups (475 milliliters)	One cup equals: 1 cup of milk or yogurt, 1½ ounces (45 grams) of natural cheese, or 2 ounces (60 grams) of processed cheese
Meat & Beans	2 ounces (60 grams)	3 to 4 ounces (85–115 grams)	One ounce equals: 1 ounce (30 grams) of meat, poultry or fish, ¼ cup cooked dry beans, or 1 egg

CHILD/ADOLESCENT NUTRITION

A healthy diet helps children grow and learn. It also helps prevent obesity and weight-related diseases, such as diabetes. Children who are overweight are more likely to develop type 2 diabetes, high blood pressure, heart disease, and other illnesses that can follow them into adulthood. Obesity in children can also lead to stress, sadness, and low self-esteem.

As children spend more time watching television and playing computer and video games, they spend less time being active. Parents play a big role in helping kids get up and get moving. Experts suggest at least 60 minutes of moderate physical activity daily for most children.

Research has shown that children who skip breakfast do not do as well in school as students who eat breakfast. A healthy breakfast includes a whole grain cereal, oatmeal, or bread with a protein such as peanut butter or a hard-boiled egg. Including whole fruit instead of fruit juice adds more vitamins, minerals, and fiber into the diet. Dairy products are acceptable as long as they are in the form of fat-free or low-fat milk, yogurt, or cheese.

When children consume a high-fat, high-sugar meal, their bodies will crash. They will become very tired and lethargic, which is not going to help them perform in school.

Lunches should include a type of whole grain, such as bread or tortillas, with a lean protein, such as tuna, turkey, or chicken. Include assortments of fruits and vegetables in various colors and sizes. Healthy beverage choices include water, fat-free or low-fat milk, or 100-percent fruit juice.

At dinner, half of a child's plate should include vegetables and fruit, one-quarter should consist of a lean protein, and one-quarter should contain whole grains, such as brown rice or whole wheat pasta.

Nutrition Guidelines for Children/Adolescents

- Offer five servings of fruits and vegetables a day.
- Choose healthy sources of protein, such as lean meat, nuts, and eggs.
- Serve whole-grain breads and cereals because they are high in fiber.
- Broil, grill, or steam foods instead of frying them.
- Limit fast food and junk food.
- Offer water and milk instead of sugary fruit drinks and sodas.
- Serve calcium-rich vegetables like broccoli, mustard greens, kale, collard greens, and brussels sprouts.
- Cook with less fat. Bake, roast, or poach foods instead of frying.
- Limit the amount of added sugar in a child's diet.
- Serve water or low-fat milk more often than sugar-sweetened sodas and fruit-flavored drinks.
- Involve the child in planning and preparing meals. Children may be more willing to eat the dishes that they help fix.
- Parents should serve as role models for their children. If children see their parents being physically active, they are more likely to be active and stay active throughout their lives.

TEEN NUTRITION

Teens may feel stressed from school, after-school activities, peer pressure, and family relationships. Many have busy schedules, that lead them to skip breakfast, buy lunch from vending machines, and grab whatever is in the refrigerator for dinner.

Healthy behaviors, like nutritious eating and regular physical activity, may help teens meet the challenges of their stressful lives. Healthy eating and regular exercise may help them feel energized, learn better, and stay alert in class. These healthy habits may also lower risks for diseases such as diabetes, asthma, heart disease, and some forms of cancer.

Many teens turn to unhealthy dieting methods to lose weight, including eating very little, cutting out whole groups of foods (like grain products), skipping meals, and fasting. Other weight-loss tactics such as smoking, self-induced vomiting, or using diet pills or laxatives can lead to health problems. Unhealthy dieting can actually cause weight gain because it slows down the metabolism.

Nutrition Guidelines for Teens

- Eat fruits and vegetables every day. Teenagers who are consuming 2,000 calories per day should aim for 2 cups of fruit and 2-1/2 cups of vegetables every day.
- Calcium helps strengthen bones and teeth. Calcium is very important, because getting enough calcium now can reduce the risk for broken bones later in life. Aim for at least three 1 cup-equivalents of low-fat or fat-free calcium-rich foods and beverages each day.
- Protein builds and repairs body tissue, like muscles and organs. Eating enough protein can help you grow strong and sustain your energy levels. Teens need five and one-half 1 ounce-equivalent of protein-rich foods each day.
- Whole-grain foods like whole-wheat bread, brown rice, and oatmeal usually have more nutrients than refined grain products. They give you a feeling of fullness and add bulk to your diet. Try to get six 1 ounce-equivalents of grains every day, with at least three 1 ounce-equivalents coming from whole-grain sources. They are also a great energy source.
- Get iron. Teen boys need iron to support their rapid growth. Most boys double their lean body mass between the ages of 10 and 17. Teen girls also need iron to support growth and replace blood lost during menstruation.

To get the iron they need, teens should eat the following foods:

- Fish and shellfish
- Lean beef
- Iron-fortified cereals
- Enriched and whole-grain breads
- Cooked dried beans and peas like black beans, kidney beans, black-eyed peas, and chickpeas/garbanzo beans
- Spinach
- Fat helps the body to grow and develop. Fat is a source of energy as well; it even keeps the skin and hair healthy. Limit your fat intake to 25 to 35 percent of your total calories each day. Limit saturated fat and trans fat, which can clog your arteries and raise your risk for heart disease. Look for words like *"shortening," "partially hydrogenated vegetable oil,"* or *"hydrogenated vegetable oil"* in the list of ingredients.

Healthier fat sources include:

- Olive, canola, safflower, sunflower, corn, and soybean oils
- Fish like salmon, trout, tuna, and whitefish
- Nuts like walnuts, almonds, peanuts, and cashews

Saturated fat is found primarily in:

- Butter
- Full-fat cheese
- Whole milk
- Fatty meats
- Coconut, palm, and palm kernel oils

Trans fat is often found in:

- Baked goods, like cookies, muffins, and doughnuts
- Snack foods, like crackers and chips
- Vegetable shortening
- Stick margarine
- Fried foods

Limit fast food and choose wisely. If you do order fast food, try these tips:

- Skip "value-sized" or "super-sized" meals.
- Choose a grilled chicken sandwich or a plain, small burger.
- Use mustard instead of mayonnaise.
- Limit fried foods or remove breading from fried chicken, which can cut half the fat.
- Order garden or grilled chicken salads with light or reduced-calorie dressings.
- Choose water, fat-free or low-fat milk instead of sweetened soda.

Research has shown that being physically active may:

- Help you control your weight, build lean muscle, and reduce your body fat.
- Strengthen your bones.
- Increase flexibility and balance.
- Reduce your risk for chronic diseases like type 2 diabetes, heart disease, and high blood pressure.
- Improve your self-esteem and mood.
- Decrease feelings of anxiety and depression.
- Help you do better in school.

Female Athlete Triad Syndrome

Girls who play sports are healthier; get better grades; are less likely to experience depression; and use alcohol, cigarettes, and drugs less frequently than girls who aren't athletes. Some girls who play sports or exercise intensely are at risk for a problem called female athlete triad. Female athlete triad is a combination of three conditions: disordered eating, amenorrhea, and osteoporosis. A female athlete can have one, two, or all three parts of the triad.

Triad Factor #1: Disordered Eating

Most girls with female athlete triad try to lose weight primarily to improve their athletic performance. The disordered eating that accompanies female athlete triad can range from avoiding certain types of food the athlete thinks are "*bad*" (such as foods containing fat) to serious eating disorders like anorexia nervosa or bulimia nervosa.

Triad Factor #2: Amenorrhea

Because a girl with female athlete triad is simultaneously exercising intensely and not eating enough calories, when her weight falls too low, she may experience decreases in estrogen, the hormone that helps to regulate the menstrual cycle. As a result, a girl's periods may become irregular or stop altogether.

Triad Factor #3: Osteoporosis

Low estrogen levels and poor nutrition, especially low calcium intake, can lead to osteoporosis. Usually, the teen years are a time when girls should be building up their bone mass to their highest levels, called peak bone mass. Osteoporosis is a weakening of the bones due to the loss of bone density and improper bone formation. Not getting enough calcium during the teen years can also have a lasting effect on how strong a girl's bones are later in life.

Signs and Symptoms of Triad Syndrome

- Weight loss
- No periods or irregular periods
- Fatigue and decreased ability to concentrate
- Stress fractures
- Muscle injuries

Signs and Symptoms of Eating Disorders

- Continued dieting in spite of weight loss
- Preoccupation with food and weight
- Frequent trips to the bathroom during and after meals
- Use of laxatives
- Brittle hair or nails
- Dental cavities (with bulimia, tooth enamel is worn away by frequent vomiting)
- Sensitivity to cold
- Low heart rate and blood pressure
- Heart irregularities and chest pain

WHAT ARE THE MOST COMMON EATING DISORDERS?

Anorexia

- avoids food at all costs
- starve themselves to the point that causes very serious weight and muscle loss from their body
- distorted body image—even when they are extremely thin they still see themselves as being overweight
- leads to a breakdown of the body's major organs, low blood pressure, malnutrition, anemia, fainting spells, seizures, infertility, and death can result from organ failure.

Bulimia

- binge eating then followed by purging (forced vomiting, excessive exercise, or laxative abuse)
- the victim has a craving for food whereas, with anorexia there is an avoidance of food

- feelings of guilt and self-disgust take over after the binge
- leads to kidney problems, rotten teeth caused by the stomach acid, fluid loss with low potassium levels; can lead to extreme weakness, near paralysis, or lethal heart rhythms, irregular periods and swallowing problems and esophagus damage

Binge Eating Disorder

- The most common of all eating disorders
- Eating large amounts of food (binge)
- Eating even when you're full
- Feeling that your eating behavior is out of control
- Eating a lot even though you're not hungry
- Frequently eating alone
- Feeling depressed, disgusted, or upset about your eating

Orthorexia Nervosa

Orthorexia, an obsession with correct eating, was defined first by Steven Bratman, M.D. Essentially, a person with orthorexia takes healthful eating to an unsafe extreme. There is nothing wrong with aiming for a healthy lifestyle and weight management, but when taken to extreme, an individual can suffer severe health and psychosocial consequences. Individuals with orthorexia often attempt to convert others to their lifestyle, actively seek out kindred dieters, and shun skeptics (Kline, 2010).

What counts as extreme?

- The individual makes ever-narrowing dietary choices.
- Planning, preparing, and eating "special" foods is a central concern.
- Resisting temptation (to stray from the regimen) dominates thoughts and acts.
- Emotional status depends on following the regimen.
- The person feels superior for following the regimen or condemns him/herself for lapses.

Treatment

- Find an eating disorder treatment specialist in your area
- **Call 1-800-931-2237, a toll-free hotline offered by the National Eating Disorders Association.**

Self-Esteem and Body Image

Self-esteem is all about how much people value themselves, the pride they feel in themselves, and how worthwhile they feel. Self-esteem is important because feeling good about yourself can affect how you act. A person who has high self-esteem will make friends easily, is more in control of his or her behavior, and will enjoy life more.

Body image is how a person feels about his or her own physical appearance.

Some teens struggle with their self-esteem and body image when they begin puberty because the body goes through many changes. Girls may feel pressure to be thin, and guys may feel like they don't look big or muscular enough. Other factors like media images can affect a person's body image, too. Family life can sometimes influence a person's self-esteem. Some parents spend more time criticizing their children and the way they look than praising them. This criticism may reduce a person's ability to develop good self-esteem. People may also experience negative comments and hurtful teasing about the way they look from classmates and peers.

Healthy Self-Esteem and Body Image

If you have a positive body image, you probably like and accept yourself the way you are. Some people think they need to change how they look or act to feel good about themselves. In reality all you need to do is change the way you see your body and how you think about yourself.

The first thing to do is recognize that your body is your own, no matter what shape, size, or color it comes in. Next, identify which aspects of your appearance you can realistically change and which you can't. Everyone (even the most perfect-seeming celeb) has things about themselves that they can't change and need to accept, like their height, or their shoe size for example.

If there are things about yourself that you want to change and can (such as how fit you are), do this by making goals for yourself. Then keep track of your progress until you reach your goal.

When you hear negative comments coming from within yourself, tell yourself to stop. Try building your self-esteem by giving yourself compliments every day. By focusing on the good things you do and the positive aspects of your life, you can change how you feel about yourself.

Resilience is the number one skill that increases self-esteem. People who believe in themselves are better able to recognize mistakes and bounce back from disappointment.

PREGNANCY

What you eat right before and during your pregnancy can affect the health of your growing baby. Even before you start trying to get pregnant, you should take special care of your health.

Getting enough folic acid is most important very early in pregnancy, usually *before* a woman knows she is pregnant. Folic acid is a B vitamin that helps prevent serious birth defects of a baby's brain or spine, called neural tube defects. Getting enough folic acid can also help prevent birth defects like cleft lip and congenital heart disease. Some breakfast cereals are enriched with 100% of the folic acid that your body needs every day.

While you are pregnant, you will need additional nutrients to keep you and your baby healthy. That does not mean, however, you need to eat twice as much. According to the American Dietetic Association (ADA), a pregnant woman needs only 300 calories a day more than she did pre-pregnancy. The ADA recommends that pregnant women eat a total of 2,500 to 2,700 calories every day.

Make sure not to restrict your diet during pregnancy either. If you do, your unborn baby might not get the right amounts of protein, vitamins, and minerals. Low-calorie diets can break down a pregnant woman's stored fat, which can lead to the production of substances called ketones. Constant production of ketones can result in a mentally retarded child.

Nutrition Guidelines during Pregnancy

- **Fruits and vegetables.** Pregnant women should try to eat 7 or more servings of fruits and vegetables combined (for example, 3 servings of fruit and 4 of vegetables) daily.
- **Whole-grains or enriched breads/cereals.** Pregnant women should eat 6 to 9 servings of whole-grain or enriched breads and/or cereals every day.
- **Dairy products.** Pregnant women should try to eat 4 or more servings of low-fat or non-fat milk, yogurt, cheese, or other dairy products every day.
- **Proteins.** Pregnant women and their growing babies need 10 grams of protein more than non-pregnant women. Pregnant women should eat 60 grams of protein every day. Two or

more 2- to 3-ounce servings of cooked lean meat, fish, or poultry without skin, or two or more 1-ounce servings of cooked meat contain about 60 grams of protein. Eggs, nuts, dried beans, and peas also are good sources of protein.

- **Don't eat uncooked or undercooked meats or fish.** These can make you sick and may harm your baby. Pregnant women should also avoid deli luncheon meats.
- **Folic acid.** Pregnant women need 400 micrograms (400 mcg) of folic acid every day to help prevent birth defects.
- **Iron.** Pregnant women need twice as much iron—30 mg per day—than other women. Some good sources of iron include lean red meat, fish, poultry, dried fruits, whole-grain breads, and iron-fortified cereals. Pregnant women need extra iron for the increased amount of blood in their bodies. Iron helps keep your blood healthy.
- **Water.** Pregnant women should drink at least 6 eight-ounce glasses of water per day. Plus, pregnant women should drink another glass of water for each hour of activity. Drinking enough water, especially in your last trimester, prevents you from becoming dehydrated. Not getting enough water can lead to premature or early labor. It also helps prevent constipation, hemorrhoids, excessive swelling, and urinary tract or bladder infections.
- **Fish and shellfish.** Fish and shellfish are a great source of protein and heart-healthy omega-3 fatty acids. But almost all fish and shellfish contain a harmful substance called mercury. Mercury mainly gets into our bodies by the fish we eat. High levels of this metal seem to be harmful to developing babies.
- Do not eat any shark, swordfish, king mackerel, or tilefish (also called golden or white snapper).
- Do not eat more than six ounces of "white" or "albacore" tuna or tuna steak each week.
- Choose shrimp, salmon, pollock, catfish, or "light" tuna because they contain less mercury.
- **Weight gain.** The American College of Obstetricians and Gynecologists (ACOG) recommends an average weight gain of 25 to 30 pounds during pregnancy. The amount of weight you should gain, however, depends on your weight before you became pregnant and your height.
- If you were underweight before becoming pregnant, you should gain between 28 and 40 pounds.
- If you were overweight before becoming pregnant, you should gain between 15 and 25 pounds.
- You should gain weight gradually during your pregnancy, with most of the weight gained in the last trimester.
- **Fetal alcohol spectrum disorders (FASD)** is a term describing a range of effects that can occur in a person whose mother drank alcohol during pregnancy. Some people with FASD have abnormal facial features and growth and central nervous system problems. People with FASD may have problems with learning, memory, attention span, communication, vision, and/or hearing. These problems often lead to problems in school and social problems. There is no safe time during pregnancy for you to drink alcohol. There is no known safe amount of alcohol to drink during pregnancy.

Caffeine is a stimulant found in colas, coffee, tea, chocolate, cocoa, and some over-the-counter and prescription drugs. Large quantities of caffeine can cause irritability, nervousness, and insomnia, as well as low birth-weight babies and miscarriages. Caffeine is also a diuretic and can rob the body of valuable water. Some studies show that drinking caffeine during pregnancy can harm the fetus. Other research suggests that small amounts of caffeine are safe.

Pregorexia

Pregorexia is a term used to describe pregnant women who exercise in excess and reduce calories in an effort to control pregnancy-related weight gain. Women who are most at risk for pregorexia are those who either had or have an eating disorder or those who either had or have a subclinical eating disorder. The pregnancy itself can trigger relapse and experiencing the following:

- A sense of loss of control
- A dissociation from her changing body
- A fear of weight gain
- A preoccupation with perfection

NUTRITION FOR OLDER ADULTS

People in the United States are living longer than ever before. Many older adults live active and healthy lives. Eating a balanced diet, keeping mind and body active, not smoking, getting regular checkups, and practicing safety habits will help you make the most of life. Studies show that a good diet in your later years reduces your risk of osteoporosis, high blood pressure, heart disease, and certain cancers.

Older people eventually face one or more problems that interfere with their ability to eat well. Social isolation is a common one. Older people who find themselves single after many years may become depressed and lose interest in preparing or eating regular meals, or they may eat only sparingly.

Chronic medical problems require many older adults to follow special diets such as a low-fat, low-cholesterol diet for heart disease, a low-sodium diet for high blood pressure, or a low-calorie diet for weight reduction. Special diets often require extra effort, but older people may instead settle for foods that are quick and easy to prepare, such as frozen dinners, canned foods, lunch meats, and others that may provide too many calories, or contain too much fat and sodium for their needs. Adverse reactions from medications can cause older people to avoid certain foods. Some medications alter the sense of taste, which can adversely affect appetite. Dementia associated with Alzheimer's and other diseases may cause older adults to eat poorly or forget to eat altogether.

Some older people have chewing difficulties and gastrointestinal disturbances, such as constipation, diarrhea, and heartburn. Because missing teeth and poorly fitting dentures make it hard to chew, older people may forego fresh fruits and vegetables, which are important sources of vitamins, minerals, and fiber. Or they may avoid dairy products, believing they cause gas or constipation. By doing so, they miss out on important sources of calcium, protein, and some vitamins.

Lack of money is a particular problem among older Americans, who may have no income other than Social Security. Lack of money may lead older people to scrimp on important food purchases—for example, perishable items like fresh fruits, vegetables, and meat because of higher costs and fear of waste.

Nutrition Guidelines for Older Adults

Researchers from Tufts University developed a Food Guide Pyramid to more accurately represent the calorie and special nutrient needs for healthy persons over the age of 70.

- Eat at least the minimum number of servings for each food group in the Food Guide Pyramid. Eat a variety of foods that are good sources of protein, vitamins, minerals, and fiber.
- Eat at least 3 servings of calcium-rich foods. Calcium and vitamin D are important to maintain bone health.

- Drink 8 cups of water as the base of the 70+ Pyramid. This is needed because of higher intake of medications and to prevent dehydration and constipation.
- Eat fiber-rich foods from grains, fruits, vegetables, dried beans, and nuts.
- Eat fortified foods with vitamin B12, calcium, and vitamin D.
- Avoid empty calories, which are foods with lots of calories but few nutrients, such as chips, cookies, soda, and alcohol.
- Pick foods that are low in cholesterol and fat, especially saturated and trans fats.

Physical activity can help reduce and control weight by burning calories. Moderate exercise that places weight on bones, such as walking, helps maintain and possibly even increases bone strength in older people. A study published in the Dec. 28, 1994, *Journal of the American Medical Association* found that intensive strength training can help preserve bone density and improve muscle mass, strength, and balance in postmenopausal women. In the study, subjects used weight machines for strength training. Regular exercise can improve the functioning of the heart and lungs, increase strength and flexibility, and contribute to a feeling of well-being.

NUTRITION ASSIGNMENT #5

1. Summarize some important nutritional guidelines for an: a) infant, b) toddler, c) adolescent, and d) teenager.

_____

_____

_____

_____

_____

_____

_____

_____

_____

_____

_____

_____

2. Describe the female triad syndrome.

_____

_____

_____

_____

_____

_____

_____

_____

_____

_____

_____

_____

3. What are the health complications from anorexia and bulimia?

_____

_____

_____

_____

_____

_____

_____

_____

_____

_____

_____

_____

_____

RESOURCES

Administration on Aging: *www.aoa.gov/eldfam/eldfam.asp*.

American Academy of Pediatrics: *www.aap.org/parents.html*

American Academy of Pediatrics Committee on Nutrition. 2001. "The Use and Misuse of Fruit Juice in Pediatrics." *Journal of Pediatrics* 107:1210–13.

American College of Obstetricians and Gynecologists: *http://www.acog.org*

American Dietetic Association: *www.eatright.org*

American Dietetic Association. 1998. *Staying Healthy—A Guide for Older Adults*. Chicago: The American Dietetic Association.

Dietary Guidelines for Americans. USDA and DHHS, 2005: *www.healthierus.gov/dietaryguidelines*

Effects of high-intensity strength training on multiple risk factors for osteoporotic fractures. A randomized controlled trial. 1994. (Dec 28) *Journal of the American Medical Association* 272 (24):1909–14.

Food and Nutrition Information Center, USDA. Agricultural Research Service: *www.nal.usda.gov/fnic*

International Food Information Council: *http://ific.org*

Kline, D. 2010. Today's Dietitian. (November) 12:11.

Konikoff, R. A. 1999. A modified food guide for people over 70 years. *Nutritional commentator, Tufts University*. (March).

The National Network for Child Care: *www.nncc.org*

President's Council on Physical Fitness and Sports: *www.fitness.gov*

Schlenker, E. D. 1998. Nutrition in aging. 3rd ed. Boston: McGraw-Hill

WeCan! Ways to Enhance Children's Activity and Nutrition: *wecan.nhlbi.nih.gov*

Weight-control Information Network: *www.niddk.nih.gov*

RESOURCE WEB SITES

www.mypyramid.gov is your access point for the U.S. Department of Agriculture's (USDA) food guidance system. This Web site contains general guidance on food and healthy eating, with tips and suggestions for making smart dietary choices. The site also features interactive tools that can customize food and calorie recommendations according to your age, gender, and physical activity level.

www.fitness.gov, run by The President's Council on Physical Fitness and Sports, provides regular updates on the Council's activities as well as resources on how to get involved in its programs.

www.girlshealth.gov, developed by the Office on Women's Health, provides girls with reliable health information on physical activity, nutrition, stress reduction, and more.

www.fns.usda.gov/tn is the USDA's Team Nutrition Web site, which focuses on the role nutritious school meals, nutrition education, and a health-promoting school environment play in helping students learn to enjoy healthy eating and physical activity.

www.nichd.nih.gov/msy is the National Institute of Child Health and Development's *Media-Smart Youth: Eat, Think, and Be Active!* program. This interactive after-school program is designed to help young people become aware of the media's influence on their food and physical activity choices.

www.cdc.gov/powerfulbones is part of the Centers for Disease Control and Prevention's (CDC) *Powerful Bones, Powerful Girls*, which is a national health campaign that provides tips on healthy eating and physical activity.

www.canfit.org, the Web site of the California Adolescent Nutrition and Fitness Program, provides resources on adolescent nutrition and body image, fitness, and more.

http://hin.nhlbi.nih.gov/portion/keep.htm is a quiz from the National Heart, Lung, and Blood Institute that tests your knowledge of how food portion sizes have changed during the last 20 years.

www.cdc.gov/nccdphp/dnpa/physical/index.htm, a site sponsored by the CDC's Division of Nutrition and Physical Activity, addresses the importance of physical activity and provides recommendations on how to get started on a fitness program. It includes links to Web sites that offer health information for teenagers.

chapter 6
Diet and Nutrition Trends

Several prominent nutritional trends are influencing consumers to buy certain foods or follow certain eating plans. This chapter will highlight some of the trendy eating plans or "diets" consumers are trying now, as well as other trends that have gained a loyal following.

GENETICALLY MODIFIED ORGANISMS (G.M.O.)

Genetically modified foods first entered the market in the early 1980s. Genetically modified organisms have had specific changes introduced into their DNA by genetic engineering techniques.

At the beginning of 2011 the United States Department of Agriculture (USDA) approved three new kinds of genetically engineered foods: alfalfa, a corn variation that produces ethanol gas, and sugar beets. What is at issue here is that the Food and Drug Administration (FDA) and the USDA will not require any of these products, or foods containing them, to be labeled as genetically altered so as not to imply that these foods are different. Until this, a consumer could choose to purchase organic foods, which by law can't contain more than 5% GMOs, to ensure that they weren't eating or were eating a minimal amount of, genetically engineered foods.

Why GMO? These products do what Americans like best: they grow fast, which means a cheaper monetary cost for all involved. They also require fewer pesticide, fertilizers, and herbicides and, not surprisingly, they may be more profitable. What's at risk, though, is potential allergic reactions and antibiotic-resistant properties of genetically altered foods. There's also the significant risk of cross-breeding and what consequences that may lead to.

What can you do? Look for organically labeled foods, but more importantly in the case of GMOs, look for the product to indicate on the label that it does not contain genetically modified organisms.

Until the American consumer realizes that good, wholesome food doesn't come cheap, things like GMOs and newer food technologies will continue to infiltrate the food supply.

ORGANIC FOOD

Organic food is produced according to certain production standards. Simply put, it is grown without the use of conventional pesticides, artificial fertilizers, human waste, or sewage sludge, and it is processed without ionizing radiation or food additives. Livestock are reared without use of antibiotics and without the use of growth hormones.

The term *natural* does not mean organic. Unfortunately, consumers confuse the two terms. Natural can refer to one or more ingredients derived from a plant or animal that's added for flavor, not nutrition. For example, mint ice cream may contain "natural flavor," in reference to the peppermint added.

Organic food production is legally regulated. Currently, the European Union, the United States, Canada, Japan, and many other countries require producers to obtain organic certification to market food as organic. Organic products are now marketed in major supermarkets across the United States, and the industry is experiencing significant annual growth.

Although most of us think of milk or eggs as being available as organic, the "organic" category now includes foods like wine and caviar. The combination of significant mass marketing and health-conscious consumers who favor foods without synthetic herbicides, pesticides, or hormones, has caused organic foods to skyrocket. In fact, in 2004, retail sales of organic foods exceeded $15 billion with more than $32 billion projected by 2009 (Hansen, 2004).

What to Look For

When buying organic foods, look for the "USDA Organic" seal. Only foods in the categories of "100% organic" and "organic" may display the USDA Organic seal. The following are definitions according to the National Organic Program of the USDA (2003).

- *100% organic:* Single ingredient foods such as a fruit, vegetable, meat, milk, and cheese (excludes water and salt).
- *Organic:* Multiple ingredient foods that are 95% to 100% organic.
- *Made with organic ingredients:* 70% of the ingredients are organic.
- *Contains organic ingredients:* Contains less than 70% organic ingredients.

Many people believe that organic food is more expensive, which, in general, is accurate. Organic food costs more than conventional food because of the laborious and time-intensive systems used by the typically smaller organic farms; however, the benefits of buying organic may offset this additional cost. Consider the following points when questioning the price of organic (*www.organic.org*):

- Organic farmers do not receive federal subsidies like conventional farmers do; therefore, the price of organic food reflects the true cost of growing.
- The price of conventional food does not reflect the cost of environmental clean-ups that we pay for through our tax dollars.
- Organic farming is more labor- and management-intensive.

Why Organic?

Today's consumer often wonders if buying organic really means anything and if it is financially "worth" it, especially given all the news about rising food costs in general. Organic food is more expensive, but when it comes to the staples of your diet, organics are a worthwhile investment, with payoffs that might surprise you.

Organic Food Has More Nutrients

There are reasonably consistent findings for higher nitrate and lower vitamin C contents of conventionally produced vegetables versus organically grown foods, particularly leafy vegetables (Williams, 2002).

Organic Food May Benefit Your Waistline

A team of European scientists found in an experiment with rats that those that ate organic food were much healthier than those that ate conventional diets. The scientists found that the organically fed rats enjoyed several health benefits, including they slept better, had stronger immune systems, and were slimmer than rats fed conventional diets (*Science Daily*, 2005).

Organic Food Allows You to Avoid Toxins

A University of Washington study analyzed pesticide breakdown products (metabolites) in preschool aged children and found that children eating organic fruits and vegetables had concentrations of pesticide metabolites six times lower than children eating conventional produce (Curl et al., 2002).

Sustainable Agriculture

In its literal sense, sustainable agriculture refers to the ability of a farm to produce food indefinitely, without causing severe or irreversible damage to the health of the ecosystem. Two key issues are biophysical (the long-term effects of various practices on soil properties and processes essential for crop productivity) and socio-economic (the long-term ability of farmers to obtain and manage resources such as labor).

By the end of World War II, food productivity increased significantly as a result of new technologies, increased chemical use, and government subsidies. These changes allowed fewer farmers with reduced labor demands to produce the majority of the food in the United States.

Although there have been positive effects as a result of these changes, there have also been negative effects. Among these are topsoil depletion, groundwater contamination, the decline of family farms, continued neglect of the living and working conditions for farm laborers, increasing costs of production, and the disintegration of economic and social conditions in rural communities (University of California Sustainable Agriculture Research and Education Program).

The concept of sustainable agriculture addresses many environmental and social concerns, but also attempts to create viable opportunities for growers, laborers, consumers, policymakers, and many others in the entire food system. The 2008 Farm Bill, which passed on June 18, 2008, afforded significant gains in organic agriculture, conservation, and renewable energy and in securing open markets and fair contracts for livestock producers (National Campaign for Sustainable Agriculture).

Locally Grown

The local food movement is a collaborative effort to build more locally based, self-reliant food economies—one in which sustainable food production, processing, distribution, and consumption is integrated to enhance the economic, environmental, and social health of a particular place (Feenstra, 2002).

One way to support and enjoy the locally grown movement is by visiting a farmers' market. Farmers' markets allow consumers to have access to locally grown, farm-fresh produce. Additionally, farmers' markets give farmers the opportunity to develop a personal relationship with their customers and cultivate consumer loyalty. There are more than 4,600 farmers' markets operating throughout the nation today. To find a farmers' market near you, visit *http://apps.ams.usda.gov/FarmersMarkets/*. In addition, the National Resources Defense Council offers a state-by-state guide of foods that are in-season in any given region of the United States at *http://www.nrdc.org/health/foodmiles/*.

The following is a list of the produce available, by season, at the USDA Farmers' Market in Washington, DC (USDA Wholesale and Farmers' Markets).

Apples: July, August, September, October, November
Apricots: June, July, August
Asparagus: May, June
Beans: May, June, July, August, September, October
Beets: June, July, August, September, October, November
Blackberries: June, July, August, September
Blueberries: June, July, August, September
Broccoli: June, July, August, September, October
Brussels Sprouts: August, September, October
Cabbage: June, July, August, September, October, November
Cantaloupes: June, July, August
Carrots: June, July, August, September, October, November
Cherries: June, July
Corn: June, July, August, September, October
Cucumbers: June, July, August
Eggplant: June, July, August, September
Flowers: June, July, August, September, October, November
Greens: May, June, July, August, September, October, November
Grapes: July, August, September, October
Herbs: May, June, July, August, September, October, November
Leeks: September, October, November
Lettuce: May, June, July, August, September
Nectarines: July, August, September
Okra: June, July, August, September
Onions: May, June, July, August, September, October
Peaches: June, July, August, September
Pears: August, September, October, November
Peas: May, June, July
Peppers: June, July, August, September, October
Plums: July, August, September, October
Potatoes: June, July, August, September, October, November
Pumpkins: October, November
Radishes: May, June, July
Raspberries: June, July, August, September, October
Rhubarb: May, June, July
Squash: June, July, August, September
Strawberries: May, June, July
Tomatoes: June, July, August, September
Turnips: July, August, September
Watermelons: July, August, September
Zucchini: June, July, August, September

FUNCTIONAL FOOD

Functional food is any fresh or processed food with a claim to have a health-promoting and/or disease-preventing property beyond the basic nutritional function of supplying nutrients. Examples include fruits and vegetables, whole grains, fortified or enhanced foods and beverages, and some dietary supplements (*International Food Information Council*, 2006). The term functional food was first introduced in Japan in the mid-1980s. Japan was the first country to formulate a specific regulatory approval process for functional foods (Hasler, 1998).

The Food and Drug Administration (FDA) regulates food products according to their intended use and the nature of claims made on the package. Consumers can have peace of mind that a governmental body is regulating functional foods, although they should not automatically assume that consuming functional foods will make them healthier, cure diseases, and allow them to live longer lives. It is true, however, that enhanced foods may be useful for those with unique nutritional needs, such as vegans, who consume no animal products and need to ensure getting certain nutrients like calcium and vitamin B12. Consumers should be aware of mega-dosing on certain nutrients when consuming a lot of functional foods. For example, if you drink calcium-fortified orange juice at breakfast, take a calcium supplement, and have a latte, you may be consuming more of this particular nutrient than your body needs.

Five types of health-related statements or claims are allowed on food and dietary supplement labels:

1. *Nutrient content claims:* Indicate the presence of a specific nutrient at a certain level.
2. *Structure and function claims:* Describe the effect of dietary components on the normal structure or function of the body.
3. *Dietary guidance claims:* Describe the health benefits of broad categories of foods.
4. *Qualified health claims:* Convey a developing relationship between components in the diet and risk of disease, as reviewed by the FDA and supported by the weight of credible scientific evidence available.

5. *Health claims:* Confirm a relationship between components in the diet and risk of disease or health condition, as approved by FDA and supported by significant scientific agreement (International Food Information Council, 2006).

A large body of credible, scientific research is needed to confirm the benefits of any particular food or component. For functional foods to deliver their potential public health benefits, consumers must have a clear understanding of and a strong confidence in the scientific criteria that are used to document health statements and claims (International Food Information Council, 2006). Still, the nutritional scientific community disagrees on the exact definition of a functional food.

What are Some Functional Foods?
- Calcium-fortified orange juice
- Plant sterols: special, fortified margarines, like Promise or Benacol
- Nutrient-enhanced salad dressings with added Omega-3 Fatty Acids
- Green tea: high antioxidant levels
- Soluble fiber: oatmeal and legumes (may help lower cholesterol levels)
- Soy protein like that found in tofu (may lower cholesterol)
- Omega-3 Fatty Acids: fatty fish, added to some pastas like Barilla Plus brand, helps decrease inflammation and cholesterol levels

- Resveratrol: reduce inflammation and help reduce heart disease risk; high antioxidants, red wine/grape juice
- Lycopene: tomatoes and processed tomato products (may reduce the risk of prostate cancer), high antioxidant level
- Probiotics: fermented dairy products with live active cultures (may help support gastrointestinal health)
- Lutein: spinach, kale, collard greens (may reduce the risk of age-related macular degeneration), high antioxidant level

FOODS THAT BURN FAT

It has been scientifically proven that some foods increase the rate at which your body burns calories. Eating these foods won't work on their own if you are not exercising and maintaining a healthy diet.

Cayenne pepper—helps you burn more calories by triggering a thermodynamic burn that lasts hours after eating, it also enhances the way cholesterol is processed by the body. It also makes you sweat and raises your heart rate, so your metabolism increases for a few hours after eating it.

Cinnamon—research conducted by the USDA has proven that as little as a ¼ teaspoon of cinnamon added to food helps your body to metabolize sugar 20 times faster and lower your body's blood-sugar levels.

Ginger—is a vasodilator, which expands the blood vessels, increases body heat and metabolism by 20%. It also detoxifies the body and stimulates circulation.

Citrus fruit—lemons, oranges, grapefruit, and limes are incredibly high in *vitamin C*, which has a fat-burning component. Start out your morning with a glass of warm water and a squeeze of lemon.

Apples and berries—contain an abundance of pectin which has a water-binding property and, when ingested, limits the amount of fat your cells absorb.

—The watery build-up that results from pectin drowns out the fat from the cells and keeps your body from absorbing it.

Soybeans—have lecithin, which helps your body to keep your cells from accumulating fat.

Bananas—contain potassium, a naturally occurring chemical that boosts your metabolism and regulates your body's water balance, also known as a natural diuretic.

EFAs—those who consume fish regularly have lower levels of a protein hormone called leptin, which has been linked to a slower metabolism and obesity. The best fish to eat are wild salmon, tuna, herring, and mackerel.

Garlic—is a natural antibiotic, and it regulates blood sugar, while increasing your metabolism. Garlic works like a thermogenic in your body, boosts your metabolism, and keeps your insulin levels low to maximize fat burning.

Low-fat dairy and protein—The International Journal of Obesity published a study in April 2005 that concluded that calcium and protein that come from low-fat dairy products actually promote weight loss and help to maintain muscle mass.

EATING PLANS

Several different eating plans or diets have gained significant popularity in the last decade.

The Atkins Diet Weight Loss Program

The Atkins Diet is the "father" of the high-protein, low-carbohydrate plans. Dr. Robert Atkins published his first version of the program in 1973. Today it continues to be a popular nutritional trend. The Atkins Diet advocates eliminating virtually all carbohydrates and promotes the consumption of protein. No more bagels or pancakes at breakfast, sandwiches at lunch, or pasta at dinner. Instead, you can consume almost endless quantities of eggs, luncheon meats, beef, and poultry. The Atkins Diet is very difficult to maintain long-term, but works if you think you can live the rest of your life bread-free and sugar-free, with very little fruit and a restricted list of vegetables from which to choose.

The plan is divided into four phases:

Phase 1: Induction

Phase 1 lasts a minimum of 14 days. During this phase, you must eat three regular-sized meals; eat liberal amounts of fat and protein; eat no more than 20 grams of carbohydrate per day; absolutely no fruit, bread, pasta, grains, starchy vegetables, or dairy other than cheese, cream, or butter; and avoid coffee, tea, and soft drinks that contain caffeine.

Foods Allowed During Phase 1:
- Protein: chicken, turkey, lean beef, fish, shellfish, lamb, pork, veal, eggs, and a variety of vegetable proteins like tofu.
- Natural fats: olive oil, safflower oil, butter, and avocado.
- Leafy greens and vegetables: Salad greens and non-starchy vegetables should make up around 12 grams of carbohydrates per day.
- Additional carbs daily including:
  - Up to 4 ounces of cheese
  - 10 to 20 olives for a quick snack
  - Half an avocado in a salad
  - An ounce of sour cream or 3 ounces of unsweetened cream in coffee
  - Up to 3 tablespoons lemon or lime juice
  - One to two servings of Atkins bars or shakes (Check the package to see which ones are right for induction [less than 5 net carbs]).

Foods Not Allowed During Phase 1:
- Added sugars and trans fats, though sucralose or saccharin as a sweeter is allowed. You may also have diet beverages that contain these sweeteners as well as sugar-free gelatin.
- High-carbohydrate foods including:
  - Starchy vegetables such as potatoes, yams, squash
  - Bread, rice, cereal, and pasta
  - Whole, reduced-fat or skim milk
  - Fruit, except for avocados, tomatoes, and olives
  - Nuts or seeds
  - Foods that combine protein and carbs: lentils, chickpeas (garbanzo beans), kidney beans, and other legumes.

Phase 2: On-going Weight Loss (OWL)

Phase 2 is the longest phase of the Atkins Diet plan. In this phase, you steadily increase your carbohydrate consumption. Each week, you add 5 grams of carbohydrate until you eventually reach a level at which you are no longer losing weight. This is called the "Critical Carbohydrate Level for Losing." More proteins and vegetables are added, as well as berries, nuts, and seeds. If a new food causes weight gain, then you must stop eating it. This phase lasts until you have only 5 to 10 more pounds to lose. Expect to spend a few months on Phase 2 if you have more than 40 pounds to lose.

Foods Allowed During Phase 2:
- Lean protein: chicken, turkey, lean beef, fish, shellfish, lamb, pork, veal, eggs, and a variety of vegetable proteins.
- Fats: olive oil, safflower oil, butter, and avocado.
- Vegetables, berries, nuts, and seeds (Just remember to stick with your daily Net Carb count each week).

Phase 3: Pre-maintenance

During Phase 3, you increase carbohydrate consumption until you lose less than 1 pound per week. You can add a piece of fruit or a starchy vegetable, a serving of brown rice, or sweet potatoes. Ideally, you should spend at least one month in this phase, preferably, two to three months.

Phase 4: Lifetime Maintenance

Phase 4 provides you with a way of eating so you stay slim for the rest of your life. A healthy amount of carbohydrates are allotted so you are able to maintain your weight without fluctuating more than 3 to 5 pounds.

Slim-Fast

Liquid diets have been around for a long time. Slim-Fast is well known for its "two shakes and a sensible dinner" slogan.

The Slim-Fast plan features two daily Slim-Fast meals: balanced shakes or meal bars along with a "sensible meal" and healthy snacks. This is essentially a low-fat, low-calorie, portion-controlled plan. A plus of this plan is that replacing meals with Slim-Fast products makes planning easier and can help take the guesswork out of food selection.

Dieters using this plan must buy a lot of the Slim-Fast products, which can be costly. In addition, the long-term use of the Slim-Fast products may become unrealistic. Obviously, a person has to like the way the products taste, or they will not stick to the plan.

The ingredients' lists of many of the Slim-Fast products are quite long and highly processed. A whole foods based diet would be preferable. It is best to save your money and learn to eat right without trendy and highly processed, expensive, packaged products.

Weight Watchers

Weight Watchers has been around since the 1960s and recognizes dieting as just one part of long-term weight management. The Weight Watchers philosophy promotes results from a healthy lifestyle, which encompasses all aspects: mental, emotional, and physical health.

Weight Watchers does not specify what you may or may not eat. The goal of Weight Watchers is to help people make healthy eating decisions and encourage them to enjoy more physical activity, thereby losing weight safely and sensibly and, most importantly, keeping it off.

The Weight Watchers program allows you to choose from one of two plans based on good, old-fashioned "calories in, calories out" advice.

The Flex Plan

This flex plan promotes the original Weight Watchers philosophy: "Eat the food you love and lose weight." No foods are prohibited; instead, each food is assigned points based on the food's calorie, total fat, and dietary fiber content.

This system guides food choices by encouraging a selection of healthy foods. Some examples are:

1 cup broccoli = 0 points
1/2 cantaloupe = 2 points
1 small bean burrito = 5 points
1 cup spaghetti with 1/2 cup marinara sauce = 6 points
1 6-ounce steak = 8 points
1 3-ounce grilled chicken breast = 3 points
1/4 cup regular creamy salad dressing = 8 points
1 slice bread = 2 points
1 ounce chocolate = 4 points
1 scoop vanilla ice cream = 4 points

Each person has a target daily points range, calculated based on his or her body weight. For example, a 5-foot-6-inch woman who weighs 180 pounds would be allotted between 22 and 27 points each day. A "points finder" helps members calibrate the points value of a recipe or a packaged product using the nutrition facts label.

The initial Weight Watchers' goal is to reduce body weight by 5 percent to 10 percent, and the ultimate weight goal is a body mass index less than 25. For those who have a lot of weight to lose, the goal is to lose in increments of 10 percent, which helps people stay motivated.

The Core Plan

The core plan is a newer approach for Weight Watchers that allows members to control calories by focusing their eating on a core list of wholesome nutritious foods, but without counting or tracking. The list includes foods from all the food groups: fruits and vegetables; grains and starches; lean meats, fish, and poultry; eggs and dairy products. The foods in this core list are low in fat and calories. An occasional treat outside the list is allowed.

The Zone Diet

The Zone Diet is a diet popularized by biochemist Barry Sears. It advocates consuming calories from carbohydrates, protein, and fat in a 40:30:30 ratio.

"The Zone" is Sears' name for proper hormone balance. He argues that when insulin levels are neither too high nor too low, and glucagon levels are not too high, specific anti-inflammatory chemicals are released. The diet claims that a 30:40 ratio of protein to carbohydrates triggers this effect, and this is called "The Zone." Sears claims that these natural anti-inflammatories are heart, and health-friendly. This "hormonally correct diet" claims lasting fat loss, greater health, peak athletic, mental, and emotional performance, as well as a longer lifespan.

The cardinal rule of the Zone Diet is to ensure that each meal and snack has the right combination of low-fat protein, "good" carbs, and a bit of fat. Meal timing is also essential to ensure adequate "medication" every four to six hours.

Ultimately, the Zone Diet is easier than the Atkins Diet in terms of restriction and maintenance. Still, some who follow the diet report feeling fatigued and find it hard to maintain.

The South Beach Diet

The South Beach Diet was created by Dr. Arthur Agatston, a cardiologist. You will be eating 3 normal-size meals and 2 snacks each day. There are basically 3 phases in the South Beach Diet.

You eat normal portion sizes in Phase 1, but all carbohydrate are restricted. This is the strictest phase in the diet and will last for 2 weeks. It emphasizes lean meats, such as chicken, turkey, fish, and shellfish. Low-Glycemic-index vegetables are allowed as well as low-fat cheese, nuts, and eggs. Dieters should expect to lose somewhere between 8 to 12 pounds.

In Phase 2, some of the banned foods are slowly introduced while weight loss continues to around 1–2 pounds per week. You should remain on it until you lost your desired amount of weight.

Phase 3 is for maintenance and should be followed for life. It is all about maintaining your desired weight with a healthy, balanced diet.

NUTRITION ASSIGNMENT #6

1. Follow one diet listed in this chapter for a few days. Describe your experiences.

_____

_____

_____

_____

_____

_____

_____

_____

_____

_____

_____

_____

_____

_____

_____

_____

_____

_____

_____

_____

_____

_____

_____

_____

_____

_____

_____

_____

_____

_____

_____

_____

2. Define organic foods and functional foods; give examples of each. Where can you purchase organic food in your neighborhood?

_____

_____

_____

_____

_____

_____

_____

_____

_____

_____

_____

_____

_____

_____

_____

_____

_____

_____

_____

_____

_____

_____

_____

_____

_____

_____

_____

RESOURCES

Curl, C. L., Fenske, R. A., Elgethun, K. 2002. Organophosphorus pesticide exposure on urban and suburban pre-school children with organic and conventional diets. *Environmental Health Perspectives*, National Institute of Environmental Sciences.

Feenstra, G. 2002. Creating space for sustainable food systems: lessons from the field. *Agriculture and Human Values* 19 (2):99–106.

Hansen, N. 2004. Organic food sales see healthy growth. Retrieved October 20, 2008: from *MSNBC.com*.

Hasler, C. M. 1998. Functional foods: their role in disease prevention and health promotion. *Food Technology* 52 (2):57–62.

International Food Information Council. November, 2006. Retrieved October 27, 2008, from: *http://www.ific.org/nutrition/functional/index.cfm*.

National Campaign for Sustainable Agriculture. Retrieved October 20, 2008, from: *http://www.sustainableagriculture.net/site/PageServer?pagename=About_Main*.

National Resources Defense Council: Eat Local. Retrieved October 20, 2008, from *http://www.nrdc.org/health/foodmiles/*.

Organic Food Standards and Labels: The Facts. National Organic Program. Retrieved October 20, 2008.

United States Department of Agriculture National Organic Program: Labeling Packaged Products, January 9, 2003.

United States Department of Agriculture Wholesale and Farmers Markets. Retrieved October 20, 2008, from: *http://www.ams.usda.gov/AMSv1.0/ams.fetchTemplateData.do?template= TemplateN&navID=WFMUSDAMarketSeasonalProduce&rightNav1=WFMUSDAMarket SeasonalProduce&topNav=&leftNav=WholesaleandFarmersMarkets&page=WFMUSDAMarket SeasonalProduce&resultType=&acct=frmrdirmkt*.

University of California Sustainable Agriculture Research and Education Program. Retrieved October 20, 2008, from: *http://www.sarep.ucdavis.edu/Concept.htm*.

University of Newcastle Upon Tyne. 2005, March 29. Organic Diet Makes Rats Healthier. *ScienceDaily*. Retrieved October 20, 2008, from: *http://www.sciencedaily.com/releases/ 2005/03/050328182123.htm*

Williams, C. M. 2002. Nutritional quality of organic food: shades of grey or shades of green? *Proceedings of the Nutrition Society* 61:19–24.

chapter 7
Dangers in Our Food Supply

Across spectrums of gender, race, age, and socio-economic status, Americans are sicker than people in other Western countries. This is in large part due to the contamination of our food supply. In the United States, more than 3,000 substances can be added to foods for the purpose of preservation, coloring, texture, increasing flavor, and more. Although each of these substances is legal to use (at least in the United States), whether or not they are all something you want to be consuming is another story all together.

Food Additives that are Common in Most Packaged Foods Can:

- Make you fat
- Give you cancer
- Cause you to get diabetes
- Give you heart disease
- Cause high blood pressure
- Cause hormone imbalances

INGREDIENTS TO AVOID

The first step in starting a healthier lifestyle is to pay attention to the ingredients in the foods you buy. If you cannot pronounce the ingredients, chances are you should not be eating them. Healthy foods should contain simple ingredients that are easily recognizable. You should also be careful about purchasing an item that has more than five to seven ingredients in it.

Cancer-Causing Ingredients

BHA is a preservative that the International Agency for Research on Cancer (IARC) classifies as a possible carcinogen; it possibly causes cancer. It may be used to preserve foods, like cereal, that come in a box, or it may be sprayed on the packaging instead. Either way it should be avoided.

Potassium bromate is in brominated flour, often found in bread. It is classified as a possible carcinogen. Most countries in the world have banned this ingredient, except for the United States and Japan.

Citrus Red No. 2, or FD&C Citrus Red No. 2, is also a possible carcinogen. Its use is limited to coloring orange skins. If you eat the orange peel or grate it to use in any foods that you make, you will be eating a chemical that possibly causes cancer.

FD&C colors are generally derived from coal tar. Coal tar is a human carcinogen. It is known to cause cancer.

Smoked foods may contain nitrosamines and polycyclic aromatic hydrocarbons (PAH), both of which can cause cancer. There is not enough information to know if smoked flavorings pose the same risk.

Most processed meats, unless you buy organic and nitrite-free, contain nitrates or nitrites, which are chemicals that are classified as probable carcinogens by the IARC. In other words, they probably cause cancer.

Processed meats include:
- Bacon
- Ham
- Sausage
- Hot dogs
- Pepperoni
- Salami
- Pastrami
- Bologna
- Deli meats, like chicken, turkey, roast beef
- Pickled vegetables that are prepared the traditional way as done in Asia

A simple general rule is to avoid as many additives as possible, especially:

- Partially hydrogenated fats
- High fructose corn syrup
- Sodium nitrite and/or nitrates
- Fake sugars
- Olestra
- Monosodium glutamate (MSG)
- Acesulfame K
- Excessive salt and sugar
- Artificial coloring

Monosodium Glutamate (MSG)

MSG is used as a flavor enhancer in many packaged foods, including soups, salad dressings, sausages, hot dogs, canned tuna, potato chips, and many more. Many consumers have experienced the ill effects of MSG, which leave them with a headache, nausea, or vomiting after eating MSG-containing foods. MSG is known as an excitotoxin which is a group of excitatory amino acids that can cause sensitive neurons to die.

According to the FDA, MSG Symptom Complex can result in:
- Numbness
- Burning sensation
- Tingling
- Facial pressure or tightness
- Chest pain
- Headache
- Nausea

- Rapid heartbeat
- Drowsiness
- Weakness
- Difficulty breathing for asthmatics

Americans associate MSG with Chinese food; however, MSG is in many more foods than Chinese food, and is listed under many other names than MSG. Some ingredient labels hide MSG under names that consumers won't recognize, such as hydrolyzed soy protein. In terms of labeling requirements, the FDA says that "monosodium glutamate" must be listed on the label only if MSG is added to a food. However, it's misleading for a manufacturer to list "No MSG" or "No Added MSG" on foods if sources of free glutamates, like hydrolyzed protein, exist. Further, items listed as "flavors," "natural flavors," or "flavorings" may not include MSG, hydrolyzed proteins, or autolyzed yeast.

MSG is found in:

- Autolyzed yeast
- Calcium caseinate
- Gelatin
- Glutamate
- Glutamic acid
- Hydrolyzed protein
- Monopotassium glutamate
- Monosodium glutamate
- Sodium caseinate
- Textured protein
- Yeast extract
- Yeast food
- Yeast nutrient

High Fructose Corn Syrup

The process for making the sweetener high fructose corn syrup (HFCS) out of corn was developed in the 1970s. Until the 1970s most of the sugar we ate came from sucrose derived from sugar beets or sugar cane. HFCS began to gain popularity as a sweetener because it was much less expensive to produce. High fructose corn syrup can be manipulated to contain equal amounts of fructose and glucose, or up to 80 percent fructose and 20 percent glucose. Thus, with almost twice the fructose, HFCS delivers a double danger compared to sugar. Today, Americans consume more HFCS than sugar. HCFS is produced by processing corn starch to yield glucose, and then processing the glucose to produce a high percentage of fructose.

HFCS is just sugar in liquid form, differing from common table sugar (sucrose) mainly in how it affects the texture of foods.

Sucrose is a double sugar made of two single sugars—glucose (50 percent) and fructose (50 percent)—stuck together. HFCS also contains glucose and fructose, but the sugars are already separated and their percentages differ slightly. Because sucrose is quickly split by digestive enzymes, the body can hardly tell them apart. The processing of sucrose involves boiling it down from sugar cane or beets, and washing, clarifying, filtering, and drying the syrup.

HFCS starts out as corn, then the starch is extracted. Enzymes are used to break down the starch into glucose and to convert some of the glucose to fructose. Then a bunch of refining, separation, and evaporation steps occur. The resulting syrup is 55 percent fructose, with the rest

composed of glucose or undigested starch pieces. The HFCS used in soft drinks has a bit more fructose   than   sucrose—
55 percent as opposed to 50 percent.

Health Dangers of HFCS

Since HFCS's widespread introduction in the 1980s North American obesity rates have skyrocketed. When HFCS is ingested, it travels straight to the liver which turns the sugary liquid into fat, and unlike other carbohydrates HFCS does not cause the pancreas to produce insulin; which acts as a hunger quenching signal to the brain. So we are eating food that gets immediately stored as fat and we don't feel full, making us eat more and more.

Aspartame (Equal, NutraSweet)

Aspartame is the artificial sweetener found in Equal and NutraSweet, along with products that contain them (diet sodas and other low-calorie and diet foods). This sweetener has been found to cause brain tumors in rats as far back as the 1970s; however, recent studies have found that even small doses increase the incidence of lymphomas and leukemia in rats, along with brain tumors. People who are sensitive to aspartame may also suffer from headaches, dizziness, and hallucinations after consuming it.

Acesulfame-K

Acesulfame-K is an artificial sweetener that is about 200 times sweeter than sugar. It's used in baked goods, chewing gum, gelatin desserts, and soft drinks. Two rat studies have found that this substance may cause cancer. Acesulfame-K also breaks down into acetoacetamide, which has been found to affect the thyroid in rats, rabbits, and dogs.

If you want to use a sweetener:

- Use the herb *stevia*
- Use brown sugar in moderation
- Use organic raw honey
- Avoid ALL *artificial sweeteners*

Avoid excessive use of *energy drinks and sports drinks* because they are loaded with sugar, sodium, and chemical additives.

Olestra

Olestra is a fat substitute used in crackers and potato chips, marketed under the brand name Olean. This synthetic fat is not absorbed by the body (instead it goes right through it) causing diarrhea, loose stools, abdominal cramps, and flatulence. Furthermore, olestra reduces the body's ability to absorb beneficial fat-soluble nutrients, including lycopene, lutein, and beta-carotene.

Sodium Nitrite (Sodium Nitrate)

Sodium nitrite (or sodium nitrate) is used as a preservative, coloring, and flavoring in bacon, ham, hot dogs, luncheon meats, corned beef, smoked fish, and other processed meats. These additives can lead to the formation of cancer-causing chemicals called nitrosamines. Some studies have found a link between consuming cured meats and nitrite and cancer in humans.

Hydrogenated Vegetable Oil (Trans Fat)

An artificial ingredient in foods, trans fat is made when manufacturers add hydrogen to vegetable oil in an effort to increase the shelf life and flavor stability of foods containing these fats. This promotes heart disease and diabetes. Trans fats are believed to be harmful because they contribute to heart disease by raising bad cholesterol and lowering good cholesterol at the same time. The Institute of Medicine has advised that consumers should eat as little trans fat as possible. You should avoid anything with these ingredients on the label, which includes some margarine, vegetable shortening, crackers, cookies, baked goods, salad dressings, bread, and more. New York is the nation's first city to ban artery-clogging artificial trans fats in all its restaurants and other food service establishments.

Food Coloring Linked to ADHD

Consumer advocates and scientists say evidence is mounting that foods with artificial dyes may play a role in the inattentiveness, hyperactivity, and impulsivity that characterize attention-deficit hyperactivity disorder.

Blue 1 and Blue 2

Blue 1, which is used to color candy, beverages, and baked goods, may cause cancer. Blue 2, found in pet food, candy, and beverages, has caused brain tumors in mice.

Red 3

Red 3 is a food coloring used in cherries (in fruit cocktails), baked goods, and candy. It causes thyroid tumors in rats, and may cause them in humans as well.

Yellow 6

As the third most often used food coloring, yellow 6 is found in many products, including baked goods, candy, gelatin, and sausages. Yellow 6 has been found to cause adrenal gland and kidney tumors, and contains small amounts of many carcinogens.

HOW CLEAN IS OUR WATER?

Roughly 70 percent of the earth's surface is covered in water. Even though water seems to be everywhere, not all of it is suitable for use as drinking water. Of all the water on earth, only 3 percent is fresh water, with much of it frozen or underground. Less than 1 percent of the water on earth can be used as drinking water. Before we drink it and before it is released back into surface waters (such as rivers and lakes), our water must go through a variety of treatment processes.

Drinking water comes from a variety of sources. Some of the water comes from water purification plants. Some comes from underground sources. Due to the diversity of the sources, the water that we drink can differ greatly in quality and healthiness. In many instances, you cannot tell if water is contaminated by taste, smell, or by how it looks. Many common pesticides, herbicides, chemicals, and cleaners are leached into our water supply.

Bottled vs. Tap Water

Bottled water is a booming industry that grosses more than $7 billion dollars a year in the United States. Up to 40 percent of bottled water is bottled tap water that may or may not have received additional treatment. The Environmental Protection Agency (EPA) regulates the quality of public water supplies; however, it has no authority over bottled water. Further, bottled water labels can be misleading and may depict mountains and streams when the water actually came from a well in an industrial facility parking lot.

Too many factors beyond our control can drastically impact our tap water quality. Pollution in the form of chemical spills, leaking fuel tanks, pesticides, cleaning fluids, weed killers, and fertilizers is just the tip of the water-contamination iceberg. Even the very chemicals that water companies add to our water to "protect" us like fluoride, chlorine, and other disinfectants can lead to health risks.

According to a survey of 42 states by the nonprofit Environmental Working Group, a research organization in Washington, D.C., water supplies across the country meet current standards set by the U.S. Environmental Protection Agency, but contain 141 chemicals that are not regulated by the agency.

Go to *www.ewg.org/tapwater/yourwater/index.php*, or contact your local water supplier and request a quality report, which will usually detail where your water comes from and exactly what is in it. Environmental groups have also voiced concerns over the huge amounts of waste and toxins created by the bottled water industry.

One of the most overlooked sources of water contamination is water pipes. The EPA reported that even safe, potable water often becomes contaminated after it leaves the municipal treatment plant. The EPA said that sediment, such as scales and microbial material (or "biofilm"), builds up inside pipe walls and leaches into the drinking water as it passes through on the way to your home. If the water's pH is low, the acidity can result in materials like iron, copper, lead, zinc, arsenic, and manganese showing up at levels well beyond state and federal drinking water standards.

In any given year, about 25 percent of beaches in the United States are under advisories or are closed at least one time because of contamination with pathogenic bacteria, viruses, or parasites. Each year, plastic waste in water and coastal areas kills up to 100,000 marine mammals, one million sea birds, and countless fish. Around 80 percent of the pollution in seas and oceans comes from land-based activities. Water pollution is caused primarily by the drainage of contaminated waters into surface water or groundwater.

Is Bottled Water Safer?

A study by the Natural Resources Defense Council, an environmental action group, found that bottled water is no safer than tap water on average, and is sometimes less safe, containing elevated levels of arsenic, bacteria, and other contaminants. Some environmentalists, shareholder activists, and church groups are targeting Coca-Cola, PepsiCo, and Nestle, the leading sellers of bottled water. Some examples include:

- The Natural Resources Defense Council, Sierra Club, and World Wildlife Federation have all urged their supporters to consume less bottled water. A 1999 NRDC study found that bottled water was no purer or safer than most tap water.
- A handful of high-end restaurants have stopped serving bottled water.

Pepsi's Aquafina, the best-selling brand, and Coke's Dasani, which is second, are made from purified tap water. In fact, the Sierra Club states that Coca Cola's Dasani and Pepsi's Aquafina are tap water coming from places like Queens, New York, and Jacksonville, Florida, with some additional treatment. Nestle, the global leader, gets most of its water from spring sources; they are sold in North America under such regional brands as Ice Mountain, Deer Park, Poland Spring, Arrowhead, Ozarka, Zephyrhills, and Calistoga.

The Food and Drug Administration has established "Standards of Identity" for bottled water sold in the United States. Here are some of the more common identities:

Artesian water—originates from a confined aquifer that has been tapped and in which the water level stands at some height above the top of the aquifer.

Fluoridated—water contains fluoride added within the limitations established in the FDA Code of Federal Regulations.

Ground water—is from an underground source that is under a pressure equal to or greater than atmospheric pressure.

Spring water—comes from an underground formation from which water flows naturally to the Earth's surface.

Well water—is taken from a hole tapping. This hole may be bored, drilled, or otherwise constructed in the ground.

Mineral water is drawn from an underground source and contains at least 250 *ppm* of dissolved salts. Whichever minerals are present are what make mineral water what it is. Some minerals that may appear in mineral water include calcium, iron, and sodium.

Sparkling water is carbonated (contains CO_2, producing the "fizz"). It can either be naturally carbonated or mechanically carbonated in a process where CO_2 is added to normal tap water.

Seltzer water is tap water that has been filtered and carbonated. Club soda is seltzer water with added mineral salts.

Sterilized water is used to make baby formula and is also drunk by people with immuno-compromised systems. It must be processed to meet FDA's requirements for commercial sterility.

Purified water has been produced by distillation, deionization, reverse osmosis, or other suitable processes. Purified water may also be referred to as "demineralized water." It can make the body very acidic.

Distilled or demineralized water is usually tap water that has been treated to remove nearly all minerals and sodium that occur naturally in water. Since distilled water is like a vacuum without any minerals, it will actually leach beneficial minerals from your body to balance it out.

How Can I Make My Water Safe?

Everyday household activities are a major contributor to polluted runoff, which is among the most serious sources of water contamination. When it rains, fertilizer from lawns, oil from driveways, paint, and solvent residues from walls and decks, and even waste from pets are all washed into storm sewers or nearby lakes, rivers, and streams—the same lakes, rivers, and streams that we rely on for drinking, bathing, swimming, and fishing.

- Don't drink water straight from lakes, rivers, streams, or springs.
- Use a water filter and store your water in glass or BPA-free or SIGG bottles.
- You may also wish to boil your water.
- Boiling is the best way to kill germs in your water.
  - Heat your water at a rolling boil for 1 minute.
  - After the boiled water cools, put it in a clean bottle or pitcher with a lid and store it in the refrigerator.
  - Use the water for drinking, cooking, or making ice.
- Water bottles and ice trays should be cleaned with soap and water before use.

Environmental Impact

Fossil Fuel Consumption

Approximately 1.5 million gallons of oil—enough to run 100,000 cars for a whole year—are used to make plastic water bottles, and transporting these bottles burns thousands more gallons of oil. In addition, the burning of the oil and other fossil fuels, which also are used to generate the energy that powers the manufacturing process, emits global warming pollution into the atmosphere.

Waste

Only about 10 percent of plastic water bottles are recycled, leaving the rest in landfills where it takes thousands of years for the materials to decompose.

BPA and Phthalates

Over the past decade, evidence has been building that a variety of pesticides, plastics, and solvents containing chemicals can alter normal development in both wild and domestic animals.

Bisphenol A (BPA) is a chemical building block that is used primarily to make polycarbonate plastic. It's also found on the linings of cans. BPA mimics estrogen, and has been linked to breast and uterine cancer, hyperactivity, and brain damage, as well as decreased testosterone levels.

Phthalates are a family of industrial chemicals that are used as plastic softeners or solvents in many different consumer products. They are found in many beauty care products, including hair spray, deodorant, nail polish, air fresheners, laundry detergent, and perfume. Studies have shown that phthalates can damage the liver, the kidneys, the lungs, and the reproductive system, especially the developing testes. Weight gain, depression of the thyroid, and fatigue have also been reported.

Look at the triangle (▲) symbol underneath your water bottle and you will see a number inside the triangle. Polycarbonate water bottles (labeled #7) contain bisphenol A (BPA), which leaches from the plastic even at room temperature and has been linked to chromosome damage and hormone disruption. These are the types of plastic Nalgene water bottles found in sports stores. #1 PET or PETE bottles (polyethylene terephthalate) may leach DEHA, a known carcinogen, if used more than once. Additionally, your water bottle that has been refilled is likely to contain potentially harmful bacteria that grow on saliva, food particles, and fecal material from unwashed hands. Many people have reported getting diarrhea from their reused water bottles. Washing bottles with hot water and detergent or a rinse with bleach will sanitize them, but also leaches harmful chemicals out of the plastic.

Relatively Safe Plastics

#1 polyethylene terephalate (PET) used only once
#2 and #4 polyethylene
5 polypropylene (catsup bottles, yogurt containers)

Unsafe Plastics

#3 V (Vinyl) or PVC is found in cooking oil bottles and clear food packaging.

Number 3 plastics may release toxic breakdown products (including pthalates) into food and drinks. The risk is highest when containers start wearing out, are put through the dishwasher, or when they are heated (including microwaves). PVC manufacturing can release highly toxic dioxins into the environment, and the materials can off-gas toxic plasticizers into your home.

#6 polystyrene (Styrofoam) is found in disposable plates and cups, meat trays, egg cartons, and carry-out containers.

Number 6 plastics can release potentially toxic breakdown products (including styrene), particularly when heated, including that insulated coffee cup.

#7 polycarbonate (Nalgene) water bottles is found in baby bottles, three- and five-gallon water bottles, and certain food containers.

A wide range of plastic resins that don't fit into the other six categories are lumped into number 7. Some are quite safe, but the ones to worry about are the hard polycarbonate varieties, as found in various drinking containers (like Nalgene bottles) and rigid plastic baby bottles. Studies have shown polycarbonate can leach bisphenol A, a potential hormone disruptor, into liquids.

Never Use:

- Food or drinks heated in plastic containers in a microwave.
- Styrofoam cups (polystyrene #6), especially for hot liquids.
- #7 polycarbonate (Nalgene) water bottles.
- Plastic baby bottles. If you must use bottles, use only glass baby bottles with silicone, not latex, nipples, or use BPA-free baby bottles.
- Do not reuse plastic water bottles.
- When buying canned foods, look for BPA-free cans.

HOW SAFE IS AMERICA'S MEAT AND FISH SUPPLY?

In the 1906 book, *The Jungle*, Upton Sinclair described slaughterhouse conditions and meat contamination so horrific that the government stepped in and created a new agency to monitor the business: the Food and Drug Administration (FDA). The public's response to this book prompted the government to pass the Meat Inspection Act in 1906. The act empowered the U.S. Department of Agriculture (USDA) to require sanitary equipment, conditions, and methods, and to ban the use of harmful chemicals and preservatives in slaughtering and packing plants. Unfortunately the story did not end happily ever after.

In 2007, there were more than 20 beef recalls in the United States, totaling 33.4 million pounds. Most were prompted by the public health threat of harmful bacteria, such as *E. coli* and *salmonella*. In February 2008, a YouTube video showed disturbing images of sick cows in a meat processing plant in California. The video showed how "downer cows"—those so injured or sick that they can't stand up—were processed and entered into the nation's food supply. Particularly troubling is that about a quarter of the recalled meat, which amounts to about 37 million pounds, went to schools and federal nutrition programs in 36 states.

Agricultural Practices

Some chickens never see a barnyard but instead spend their short lives in a windowless warehouse where every aspect of the birds' environment is controlled to make them grow as quickly and inexpensively as possible. It is not uncommon to have as many as 80,000 birds per warehouse. This is too large a flock to create any sense of social (or pecking) order among the chickens, so they go crazy pecking each other, sometimes to death. It is also a common practice to debeak the birds to make life easier in the crowded warehouse.

These birds grow so fast and so fat that many develop skeletal disorders that prevent them from walking or standing. Their life span averages only about two months instead of an expected 15 to 20 years for a free-roaming chicken. Because their laboratory feed is loaded with antibiotics, sulfa drugs, arsenic compounds, growth hormones, and pesticides, these birds are not exactly a picture of health. Dietary deficiencies can result in retarded growth, deformities, blindness, and disease.

After birth, most bulls are castrated and dehorned. Cattle are then allowed to roam on the range for six months to a year until they are sent off to a standing-room-only feedlot where they are fattened up for slaughter. To obtain the optimum weight in the least amount of time, feedlot managers implant time-release anabolic steroid pellets in the cattle's ears, which will increase their hormone levels two to five times. Routine use of human antibiotics in animal production may produce resistant strains of bacteria which can be transferred to humans. Besides growth hormones and antibiotics, pesticide and herbicide residues are another potential danger to the meat eaters of America.

The Slaughterhouse

Working conditions in a slaughterhouse are far from ideal. Low-paid workers suffer a high rate of personal injury and disability, the second highest of any occupation in the United States. Sixty to seventy chickens may be checked by one person per hour. Workers are cutting up to 300 cows an hour, working long hours with few breaks. Many plants have an employee turnover rate of more than 40 percent, resulting in too many untrained workers. Because union membership is discouraged and workers are worried about job security, nothing is done to fix dangerous working environments.

Mercury

Mercury occurs naturally in the environment and can also be released into the air through industrial pollution. Mercury falls from the air and can accumulate in streams and oceans which is turned into methylmercury in the water. Fish absorb the methylmercury as they feed in these waters and, as a result, it accumulates in their tissues. In America, 1 in 6 children born every year has been exposed to mercury levels so high that he or she is potentially at risk for learning disabilities, motor skill impairment, and short-term memory loss.

Fish and shellfish are an important part of a healthy diet. Fish and shellfish contain high-quality protein and other essential nutrients, are low in saturated fat, and contain omega-3 fatty acids. A well-balanced diet that includes a variety of fish and shellfish can contribute to heart health; however, some fish and shellfish contain higher levels of mercury that may harm an unborn baby or young child's developing nervous system. The risks from mercury in fish and shellfish depend on the quantity and types of seafood consumed. The Food and Drug Administration (FDA) and the Environmental Protection Agency (EPA) advise women who may become pregnant, pregnant women, nursing mothers, and young children to avoid some types of fish and eat fish and shellfish that are lower in mercury.

1. Avoid shark, swordfish, king mackerel, and tilefish because they contain high levels of mercury.
2. Eat up to 12 ounces (2 average meals) a week of a variety of fish and shellfish that are lower in mercury.
    - Five of the most commonly eaten fish that are low in mercury are shrimp, canned light tuna, wild salmon, pollock, and catfish.

To review a list of fish to consume or avoid, visit: *http://www.mbayaq.org/cr/cr_seafoodwatch/download.asp*

Best Choices

Arctic char (farmed)
Barramundi (U.S. farmed)
Catfish (U.S. farmed)
Clams, mussels, oysters (farmed)
Clams: softshell/steamers (wild)
Crab: Dungeness
Croaker: Atlantic
Halibut: Pacific
Herring: Atlantic/sardines
Lobster: Spiny (U.S.)
Pollock (Alaska wild)
Salmon (Alaska wild)
Scallops: Bay (farmed)
Squid: Longfin (U.S.)
Striped bass (farmed or wild*)
Sturgeon, caviar (farmed)
Swordfish (Canada, U.S. harpoon, handline)
Tilapia (U.S. farmed)
Trout: Rainbow (farmed)
Tuna: Albacore (U.S., British Columbia troll/pole)
Tuna: Skipjack (troll/pole)

Good Alternatives

Basa, swai (farmed)
Black sea bass
Bluefish
Clams: Atlantic surf, hard, ocean
Quahog (wild)
Crab: Blue, Jonah, King (U.S.), Snow
Crab: Imitation/surimi
Haddock (hook and line)
Hake: Silver, red, and offshore
Lobster: American/Maine
Mahi mahi/dolphinfish (U.S.)
Oysters (wild)
Scallops: Sea (Canada and Northeast)
Scup/porgy
Shrimp: Northern
Shrimp (U.S. farmed or wild)
Squid
Swordfish (U.S. longline)
Tilefish (Mid-Atlantic)
Tuna: Bigeye, yellowfin (troll/pole)
Tuna: canned light, canned-white/albacore

Avoid

Chilean seabass/toothfish
Cod: Atlantic
Crab: King (imported)
Dogfish (Atlantic)
Flounders, soles (Atlantic)
Haddock (trawled)
Hake: White
Halibut: Atlantic
Mahi mahi/dolphinfish (imported)
Monkfish
Orange roughy
Salmon (farmed, including Atlantic)
Scallops: Sea (Mid-Atlantic)
Sharks and skates
Shrimp (imported farmed or wild)
Snapper: Red
Sturgeon, caviar (imported wild)
Swordfish (imported)
Tilefish (Southeast)
Tuna: Albacore, bigeye, yellowfin
Tuna: Bluefin

Source: www.oceansalive.org/eat.cfm.

What Can We Do?

If we choose to include meat in our diet, then how can we ensure that we are eating the safest food possible? Raising our own chickens or becoming vegetarians may be excellent alternatives. If that is not an option, consider buying naturally raised or organic meat and poultry. USDA ratings such as "prime" and "choice" refer to the marbling or fat content of the meat, not the quality. If you can't find naturally raised poultry or your grocer will not order it, look for kosher poultry, which is processed and handled according to kosher requirements.

Kosher laws are stricter than USDA standards, when it comes to the health of animals that can be eaten. They prohibit, for example, using cows with broken bones or animals that are visibly sick. The laws strictly dictate how the animals are fed, killed, and processed. Like organic meat and poultry, kosher meats and poultry are hormone-free.

The USDA approved four categories of organic labels, based on the percentage of organic content.

1. **100 Percent Organic** may carry the USDA Organic Seal.
2. **Organic** requires at least 95 percent of content to be organic by weight (excluding water and salt) to carry the USDA Organic Seal.
3. **Made with Organic** requires at least 70 percent of content to be organic and the front product panel to display the phrase "Made with Organic," followed by up to three specific ingredients (may not display the new USDA Organic seal).

4. **Less than 70% of content is organic** and may list only those ingredients that are organic on the ingredient panel with no mention of organic on the main panel (may not display the new USDA Organic seal).

Reading the stickers found on produce is an easy way to find organic fruits and vegetables. A 5-digit number beginning with 9 means it was grown organically. A 4-digit number means the food was conventionally grown. For example, the sticker on an organic apple would read "93012." A conventional one would say "4011" (Organic Trade Association).

Be careful not to cross-contaminate by spreading raw meat juices onto knives and cutting boards. Most bacteria, unlike chemical residues, will die when cooked thoroughly so forget about those medium-rare burgers on the grill (the grill and the microwave both cook unevenly). Ground meat is especially high-risk because it can be a combination of around-the-world beef or old beef mixed with fresher beef.

Reducing Risk

The EPA offers the following suggestions:

- Wash and scrub all fresh fruits and vegetables under running water or using a vegetable wash.
- Peel fruits and vegetables when possible.
- Discard the outer leaves of leafy vegetables.
- Trim fat from meat and skin from poultry. Pesticide residue can collect in fat.
- Eating a variety of foods from a variety of sources will reduce the likelihood of repeated exposure to a single pesticide.

The Environmental Working Group has created a ranking of produce by pesticide residue to help you make better choices (See table on page 122).

FOODBORNE ILLNESS

A foodborne illness is a disease carried or transmitted to people by food. Food poisoning, on the other hand, refers to the actual point in time when a food is contaminated. Each year, millions of people are affected by foodborne illness, although the majority of cases are not reported. In fact, the Centers for Disease Control (CDC) estimates 76 million cases of foodborne illness occur yearly in the United States. Among the more serious cases each year, 325,000 require hospitalization and 5,000 result in death (www.cdc.gov).

Am I At Risk For Foodborne Illness?

Anyone who eats food is theoretically at risk of developing foodborne illness. However, there are certain populations, also known as *high-risk populations*, who have a higher risk of contracting a foodborne illness than others, sometimes with serious results.

They include:

- **Infants and preschool-age children:** Young children are at a higher risk because they have not yet built adequate immune systems.
- **Elderly people:** Almost opposite of young children, older folks' immunity is on the decline and weakening with age. Also, their sense of taste and smell is not as strong.
- **Pregnant women:** A pregnant woman is at higher risk for foodborne illness and should avoid certain foods such as: deli meats, soft cheese, shellfish, raw sprouts, or undercooked meats and poultry.

The Full List: 45 Fruits and Vegetables

Rank	Fruit and Vegetable	Score
1 (worst)	Peaches	100 (highest pesticide load)
2	Apples	96
3	Sweet bell peppers	86
4	Celery	85
5	Nectarines	84
6	Strawberries	83
7	Cherries	75
8	Lettuce	69
9	Grapes (imported)	68
10	Pears	65
11	Spinach	60
12	Potatoes	58
13	Carrots	57
14	Green beans	55
15	Hot peppers	53
16	Cucumbers	52
17	Raspberries	47
18	Plums	46
19	Oranges	46
20	Grapes—domestic	46
21	Cauliflower	39
22	Tangerines	38
23	Mushrooms	37
24	Cantaloupe	34
25	Lemons	31
26	Honeydew melon	31
27	Grapefruit	31
28	Winter squash	31
29	Tomatoes	30
30	Sweet potatoes	30
31	Watermelon	25
32	Blueberries	24
33	Papaya	21
34	Eggplant	19
35	Broccoli	18
36	Cabbage	17
37	Bananas	16
38	Kiwi	14
39	Asparagus	11
40	Sweet peas—frozen	11
41	Mango	9
42	Pineapples	7
43	Sweet corn—frozen	2
44	Avocado	1
45 (best)	Onions	1 (lowest pesticide load)

Courtesy of the Environmental Working Group, Washington, D.C.

- *People taking certain medications:* Ingesting certain medications such as immunosuppressants (for diseases such as HIV/AIDS, cancer, lupus, etc.) and antibiotics increase susceptibility to pathogens present on food.
- *People with chronic illness:* Anyone who has just had major surgery, who is an organ donor/recipient, or those with illnesses like diabetes have a higher likelihood of contracting a foodborne illness.

Because these groups are of particular concern for contracting foodborne illness, it is especially important that they eat foods that are kept cold and are cooked to the appropriate internal temperature.

Riskiest Foods

According to the Food and Drug Administration's Food Code, a model used by local, state, and federal regulators to develop or update their own food safety regulations, potentially hazardous foods include: *(www.fda.gov)*

- Milk and milk products
- Meats: beef, lamb, pork
- Poultry
- Eggs
- Raw sprouts
- Shellfish and crustaceans
- Fish
- Cooked potatoes
- Heat-treated, plant-based foods like rice or beans
- Tofu or textured soy protein
- Sliced melons
- Garlic-and-oil mixtures

How Food Becomes Unsafe

Cases of foodborne illness typically involve several factors. Three common factors that contribute to its onset include: time-temperature abuse, poor personal hygiene, and cross contamination.

Keep Hot Foods Hot and Cold Foods Cold!

For microorganisms to grow and multiply, they need the right temperature. If potentially hazardous foods are kept in the temperature danger zone, which is between the temperatures of 41 to 135 degrees Fahrenheit, for four hours or longer, microorganisms can grow to levels high enough to make someone ill. Therefore, foods, especially potentially hazardous foods, should either be kept cold, cooked thoroughly, and then kept hot, if necessary (on a hot buffet, for example).

Dirty Hands = Dirty Food!

Hand washing is one of the most important things that you can do to avoid foodborne illness. Coughing, sneezing, scratching, or picking your face all can contaminate food. To avoid contracting foodborne illness due to poor personal hygiene, insist food handlers wear gloves while preparing your food, hand wash prior to eating, and encourage friends and family to hand wash when eating together. A simple rinse will not do the job. Proper hand washing should last for roughly 20 seconds, or long enough to sing, "Happy Birthday" song two times.

Using warm water and soap, create a lather and scrub under nails, in between fingers, and on backs of hands. Next, rinse and using a paper towel, turn off the water faucet. Finally, dry hands on unused portion of the paper towel.

Microorganisms Can Move from Surface to Surface—Avoiding Cross-Contamination

Cross-contamination results when microorganisms are transferred from one surface to another. This is a major contributing factor behind food-borne illness that you might least expect. If you are using utensils or a cutting board when working with meat, it's very important to NOT cut vegetables or anything else because of the risk of cross-contamination. Use a separate board for meat and be careful to use different utensils.

Steps You Can Take to Avoid Contamination

- Use color-coded cutting boards in your kitchen: red for meats, yellow for poultry, white for fish, and green for produce.
- Avoid rinsing meat/poultry/fish prior to cooking. The cooking process alone will destroy any pathogens present. Rinsing allows the opportunity for contaminated water to splash or cross-contaminate on kitchen surfaces.
- After handling raw meat/poultry/fish, wash your hands. Let's say that you have placed raw chicken breasts in a pan to bake. You open the oven and place the pan on a rack to cook. If you did not wash your hands after handling the raw chicken, you have now contaminated the handle of the oven door.
- Have plenty of clean cooking utensils on hand while cooking. Let's say that you are not certain if a piece of meat is completely cooked. And, although you plan to use a thermometer, you want to cut into it to see what color the inside meat is. Once finished, you lay the fork and knife you used on the countertop. Now, not only is the countertop contaminated, but so are the utensils.
- Finally, remember that a food can be cross-contaminated even after it is cooked! Let's say that you remove cooked chicken breasts from the oven. You place them on the counter on a plate to cool for a few minutes. They are a little cooler now, so you begin cutting them into cubes for a chicken salad you are making. While you are cutting though, you scratch an itch on the side of your nose and then finish cutting the remainder of the cooked chicken. Because of the seemingly harmless scratch on the nose, you have now cross-contaminated any microorganisms that might have been present there, such as Staphylococcus.

What Are Foodborne Disease Outbreaks and Why Do They Occur?

The Centers for Disease Control and Prevention (CDC) defines an *outbreak* of foodborne illness as when a group of people consume the same contaminated food and *two or more* of them develop the same illness. It may be a group that ate a meal together somewhere, or it may be a group of people who do not know each other at all, but who all happened to buy and eat the same contaminated item from a grocery store or restaurant.

The CDC identifies that many outbreaks are local in nature. They are recognized when a group of people realize that they all became ill after a common meal, and someone calls the local health department. This type of local outbreak might follow a catered meal at a reception, a pot-luck supper, or eating a meal at an understaffed restaurant on a particularly busy day. However, outbreaks are increasingly being recognized that are more widespread, affect persons in many different places, and are spread out over several weeks.

Some of the Most Common Foodborne Diseases

According to the CDC, the most commonly recognized foodborne illnesses are those caused by the bacteria Campylobacter, Salmonella, and E. coli O157:H7, and by a group of viruses called calicivirus, also known as the Norwalk and Norwalk-like viruses.

Campylobacter is a bacterial pathogen that can cause fever, diarrhea, and abdominal cramps. It is the most commonly identified bacterial cause of diarrheal illness in the world. These bacteria live in the intestines of healthy birds, and most raw poultry meat has Campylobacter on it. Eating undercooked chicken, or other food that has been cross-contaminated with juice drippings from raw chicken, is the most frequent source of this illness.

Salmonella is also a bacterium that is widespread in the intestines of birds, reptiles, and mammals. It can spread to humans via a variety of different foods of animal origin. The illness it causes, salmonellosis, typically includes fever, diarrhea, and abdominal cramps. In persons with poor underlying health or weakened immune systems, it can invade the bloodstream and cause life-threatening infections.

E. coli O157:H7 is a bacterial pathogen that has a reservoir in cattle and other similar animals. Human illness typically follows consumption of food or water that has been contaminated with microscopic amounts of cow feces. The illness it causes is often a severe and bloody diarrhea and painful abdominal cramps, without much fever. In 3 to 5 percent of cases, a complication called hemolytic uremic syndrome (HUS) can occur several weeks after the initial symptoms. This severe complication includes temporary anemia, profuse bleeding, and kidney failure.

Calicivirus, or Norwalk-like virus, is an extremely common cause of foodborne illness, though it is rarely diagnosed, because the laboratory test is not widely available. It causes an acute gastrointestinal illness, usually with more vomiting than diarrhea that resolves within two days. Unlike many foodborne pathogens that have animal reservoirs, it is believed that Norwalk-like viruses spread primarily from one infected person to another. Infected kitchen workers can contaminate a salad or sandwich as they prepare it, if they have the virus on their hands. Infected fishermen have contaminated oysters as they harvested them.

For automatic notification of recall updates, visit the USDA's Web site at:
http://www.fsis.usda.gov/Fsis_Recalls/index.asp

NUTRITION ASSIGNMENT #7

1. Consider the following scenario.

   It's a beautiful day and you and your friends want to have a backyard barbeque. You all decide to hit the grocery store and stock up on your favorite grilling foods: ribs, burgers, and hot dogs. You also pick up some tomatoes and lettuce that the cook sliced up and potato salad with mayo. You noticed that the chef had only 1 pair of tongs—to pick up the raw meat and the buns. The food tasted great, the party was fun, and everyone had a good time. Later that night, however, you feel horrible. You've got diarrhea, vomiting, and abdominal pain. What foodborne illness do you suspect and how could it have happened?

   _____

   _____

   _____

   _____

   _____

   _____

   _____

   _____

   _____

   _____

   _____

   _____

   _____

   _____

   _____

   _____

   _____

   _____

   _____

   _____

   _____

2. How would you advise your friends to have a safe barbeque in order to avoid the spread of foodborne illness?

_____

_____

_____

_____

_____

_____

_____

_____

_____

_____

_____

_____

3. Describe the meaning of the different triangular numbers on the bottom of bottles.

_____

_____

_____

_____

_____

_____

_____

_____

_____

_____

_____

_____

_____

RESOURCES

American Journal of Clinical Nutrition. November 2002, 76 (5):911–22.

Appleton, Nancy, PhD. Fructose is No Answer For a Sweetener: *http://www.mercola.com/ 2002/jan/5/fructose.htm*.

Beatrice Trum Hunter. Confusing Consumers About Sugar Intake. *Consumer's Research* 78, no 1 (January 1995): 14–17.

Bryan, F. L. 1982. Diseases transmitted by foods. Atlanta: Centers for Disease Control.

Centers for Disease Control and Prevention, U.S. Department of Agriculture, Food and Drug Administration: *www.cdc.gov/ncidod/dbmd/diseaseinfo/*.

Center for Science in the Public Interest: *www.cfsan.fda.gov/~dms/*.

Centre for Science and Environment: *www.cseindia.org*

Environmental Protection Agency. Local Drinking Water Reports: *www.epa.gov/safewater/ dwinfo.htm*

Environmental Protection Agency: Fish advisory 2007: *http://www.epa.gov/waterscience/fish/advice/ factsheet.html*

Environmental Working Group: *www.ewg.org*

Fallon, Sally and Mary Enig. 2001. *Nourishing Traditions*. Washington DC: New Trends Publishing, p. 23.

Food and Drug Administration (FDA) Food Code: *http://www.cfsan.fda.gov/~dms/fc05-toc.html*

Fortune Magazine. The safety of bottled water: *http://money.cnn.com/2007/04/24/news/economy/ pluggedin_gunther_water.fortune/*

Glennon, John. 2002. *Water Follies, Groundwater Pumping and the Fate of America's Fresh Waters*. Island Press.

Hallfrisch, Judith. Metabolic Effects of Dietary Fructose. *FASEB Journal* 4 (June 1990): 2652–260.

Hartford Advocate News, August 28, 2003.

Howard, Brian. Message in a Bottle. *E Magazine*, Sept/Oct 2003: *www.emagazine.com*

Natural Resource Defense Council: *http://www.nrdc.org/default.asp*.

Natural Resources Defense Council: *www.nrdc.org/water/drinking/bw/bwinx.asp*

Nestle, M. *What to Eat*. May 2006. Farrar, Straus and Giroux, LLC.

New York Times Magazine article "Power Steer," March 31, 2002.

NSF Bottled Water program: *www.nsf.org*.

Organic Trade Association: *http://www.ota.com*

Outbreak Alert! 2005. Center for Science in the Public Interest: *http://www.cspinet.org/foodsafety/*

PBS/Point of View Borders: *www.pbs.org/pov/borders/2004/water*

Schlosser, E. *Fast Food Nation*. Jan. 2001. by Mifflin.

Sinclair, U. *The Jungle*. Feb 1906. Doubleday, Jabber & Company.

United States Department of Agriculture (USDA): *http://www.fsis.usda.gov/Fsis_Recalls/index.asp*

chapter 8
Obesity and Weight Management

As Americans, we hear a lot about being "overweight" and "obese." In fact, for the first time in several decades, obesity is the *second* leading cause of preventable death in the United States, and is close to trading places with tobacco use, which is the *first* leading cause of preventable death in the United States.

Despite efforts to deal with increasingly sedentary lifestyles, Americans are, for the most part, getting fatter. Today, 65 percent of American adults over age 20 are overweight or obese, which is a pretty scary statistic. A cost of $250 billion a year is estimated for medical treatment and lost productivity from obesity and increased risk for heart disease, stroke, high blood pressure, and some forms of cancer. Obesity in our children and teens is of special concern, because an estimated one of every three kids in America today is overweight. Time spent watching television, playing video games, or sitting at the computer contributes to the problem, as do the cutbacks in physical education programs at many schools.

How Did So Many People Get So Heavy?

Most of us are eating more calories than we are burning. The problem of an overweight population comes from a combination of factors:

- Increasing portion sizes,
- More processed foods with fewer nutrients, and
- A more sedentary lifestyle.

We are eating more food. Portions have increased dramatically in the last 20 years. Bigger portions mean that we have to work a lot harder to burn the extra calories that those larger portions add.

We are eating a lot of foods that do not provide many nutrients. We are also consuming more added sugars, which is found in carbonated drinks, fruit drinks, sports beverages, and processed foods. Evidence suggests that drinking calorie-containing beverages may not make you feel full, which can lead you to eat and drink more than you need, adding even more calories to your diet.

We are eating out more often than ever before. The danger in eating out is that many types of food eaten away from home, including fast-food and prepared meals you buy at the grocery store, are high in saturated fat, trans fat, cholesterol, added sugars, and sodium. They also can be low in fiber and vitamins and minerals. In addition, people tend to eat larger portions when eating out.

We are less active. Current estimates indicate that more than half of the adults in the United States do not engage in any regular physical activity at all. As we spend more of our free time in front of televisions, computers, and video games, we are more likely to put on pounds. Our increasingly sedentary lifestyles are putting us at risk for serious health problems, including cardiovascular disease, type 2 diabetes, osteoporosis, depression, and breast and colon cancer.

- More than 50 million Americans are currently on a diet, with roughly 5 percent losing weight over the long term.
- Obesity among adults has more than doubled since 1980.
- Less than one-third of Americans meet the federal recommendations to engage in at least 30 minutes of moderate physical activity most days of the week, and 40 percent of adults engage in no physical activity at all.

MEASURING OVERWEIGHT AND OBESITY

There are a few different ways to assess whether or not a person is overweight or obese. Many people rely on a traditional scale at home or at the doctor's office, but in some cases, these numbers can be misleading.

Height and Weight Charts

Height and weight tables were originally developed and heavily used by life insurance actuaries. An actuary determines a person's eligibility for insurance based on different health factors, weight being one of them. You can imagine the slight conflict of interest. In other words, when a huge insurance company creates a height-weight table, it is in its best financial interest to establish the weight ranges on the low end. Why is this? It means because you do not meet the strict weight requirements, you must pay more money to be insured.

Waist Circumference

Waist circumference is defined as the perimeter around your natural waist, where your belly button falls, not your hips. Assessing this number provides clues about a person's health that charts and tables cannot. Most importantly, it indicates where you are carrying any excess weight. People tend to fall into one of two categories:

1. Pears: *Or*   2. Apples:

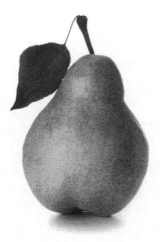

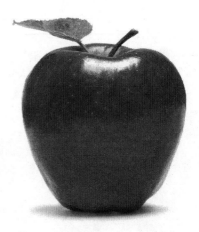

© Subbotina Anna, 2011. Used under license from Shutterstock, Inc.

© Alex Staroseltsev, 2011. Used under license from Shutterstock, Inc.

In general, men tend to be apples, whereas women tend to be pears. Once a woman hits menopause, however, she may start to accumulate body fat through the abdominal region and have more of an apple appearance instead of a pear. This is due in large part to the decrease in estrogen, which dictates where fat is stored.

What Does It Mean To Be An *Apple* Or A *Pear*?

Pears tend to accumulate any excess body fat in the hip, buttock, and thigh region whereas apples tend to accumulate it through the abdominal area. As it relates to health, it is always preferable to store excess body fat in the hip, buttock, and thigh region rather than the abdominal area. Why is this?

By the time your tailor's tape says your waistline is larger than 39 inches, you may already be on the road to diabetes or heart disease. This holds true for both men and women (Wahrenberg, 2005). Excessive abdominal fat is serious because it places you at greater risk for developing obesity-related conditions, such as type 2 diabetes, high blood cholesterol, high triglycerides, high blood pressure, and coronary artery disease.

More specifically, it is recommended that men maintain a stricter waist circumference of 35″ or less and women maintain a waist circumference of 32.5″ or less (Roizen & Oz, 2006).

Why? Wahrenberg's research found that half of all men and women with waistlines of one meter or more—that's 39.37″ or more in the United States—already have insulin resistance, where the body's cells are less responsive to the hormone insulin. On the other hand, very few people with smaller waists have developed this dangerous condition.

How To Measure Your Waist Size and Waist-to-Hip Ratio

To measure your waist size (circumference), place a tape measure around your bare abdomen above your hip bones around your belly button. Be sure that the tape is snug, but does not compress your skin, and is parallel to the floor. Relax, exhale, and measure your waist.

Remember, where you carry body fat is just as important as how much you carry. People who tend to accumulate fat around the waist (apple shape) have a higher risk of heart disease, diabetes, and high blood pressure than those who carry excess weight on the hips and thighs (pear shape).

In addition to measuring your waist circumference, you can calculate your waist-to-hip ratio (WHR). This is another way to determine if the weight in your abdomen exceeds that of your thighs.

WHR is the measurement of your waist divided by the measurement of your hips. Measure your waist at the level of your belly button as instructed above. A WHR greater than 1 for men and 0.8 for women is considered unfavorable.

Body Mass Index (BMI)

Today, most physicians and other health professionals rely on a type of measurement called body mass index (BMI). Body mass index is a method of measuring a person's *degree* of overweight or obesity. It is thought to be a more sensitive indicator than traditional height-weight charts (Drummond & Brefere, 2004).

To determine your BMI, you must know your weight in pounds and your height in inches. For example, a person who is 5′6″ (66″) and weighs 136 lbs. has a BMI of 22 (see the following chart).

BMI	19	20	21	22	23	24	25	26	27	28	29	30	31	32	33	34	35
Height (inches)						Body Weight (pounds)											
58	91	96	100	105	110	115	119	124	129	134	138	143	148	153	158	162	167
59	94	99	104	109	114	119	124	128	133	138	143	148	153	158	163	168	173
60	97	102	107	112	118	123	128	133	138	143	148	153	158	163	168	174	179
61	100	106	111	116	122	127	132	137	143	148	153	158	164	169	174	180	185
62	104	109	115	120	126	131	136	142	147	153	158	164	169	175	180	186	191
63	107	113	118	124	130	135	141	146	152	158	163	169	175	180	186	191	197
64	110	116	122	128	134	140	145	151	157	163	169	174	180	186	192	197	204
65	114	120	126	132	138	144	150	156	162	168	174	180	186	192	198	204	210
66	118	124	130	136	142	148	155	161	167	173	179	186	192	198	204	210	216
67	121	127	134	140	146	153	159	166	172	178	185	191	198	204	211	217	223
68	125	131	138	144	151	158	164	171	177	184	190	197	203	210	216	223	230
69	128	135	142	149	155	162	169	176	182	189	196	203	209	216	223	230	236
70	132	139	146	153	160	167	174	181	188	195	202	209	216	222	229	236	243
71	136	143	150	157	165	172	179	186	193	200	208	215	222	229	236	243	250
72	140	147	154	162	169	177	184	191	199	206	213	221	228	235	242	250	258
73	144	151	159	166	174	182	189	197	204	212	219	227	235	242	250	257	265
74	148	155	163	171	179	186	194	202	210	218	225	233	241	249	256	264	272
75	152	160	168	176	184	192	200	208	216	224	232	240	248	256	264	272	279
76	156	164	172	180	189	197	205	213	221	230	238	246	254	263	271	279	287

Source: National Heart, Lung, and Blood Institute (NHBLI) of the U.S. Department of Health and Human Services

Understanding Your BMI

There are four main BMI categories:

1. **Underweight** = <18.5
2. **Normal weight** = 18.5 to 24.9
3. **Overweight** = 25 to 29.9
4. **Obesity** = BMI of 30 or greater

Overweight Versus Obese

What is the difference between being overweight and being obese? Overweight and obesity are both labels for ranges of weight that are greater than what is generally considered healthy for a given height. The terms also identify ranges of weight that have been shown to increase the likelihood of certain diseases and other health problems (Centers for Disease Control and Prevention, 2007).

For adults, overweight and obesity ranges are determined by using weight and height to calculate body mass index. An adult who has a BMI between 25 and 29.9 is considered overweight whereas an adult who has a BMI of 30 or higher is considered obese.

If you have been thinking about your current weight, it may be because you've noticed a change in how your clothes fit. Or maybe you have been told by a health care professional that you have high blood pressure or high cholesterol and that your weight could be a contributing factor. The first step is to determine whether or not your current weight is healthy. BMI is just one way to determine whether your weight is a healthy one.

Body Fat Percentage

One of the best ways to really determine your "fatness" is to have your body composition assessed. The human body is made up of water (roughly 60 percent), bone mineral, organs and other tissue/viscera, muscle, and fat. When a person steps on a scale, the number he or she sees is greatly influenced by factors such as water retention, hormone fluctuation, and the weight of the fecal matter in the intestines. If you are going to weigh yourself, do so no more than one time per week (unless your doctor instructs otherwise), after a bowel movement, and before eating or drinking anything.

Have you ever noticed how two people whose heights and weights are the same can look so different? For example, let's say that in front of you stand two women who have the exact same statistics:

- Both are 5'8"
- Both are 35 years old
- Both weigh 145 lbs.
- Both have a medium bone frame

When you look at both of these women, even though they share all of the above statistics, they look very different. One of the women looks much smaller than the other. What's going on?

The answer is that they have different body composition. At this point, it is important to recognize that muscle and adipose (fat) are two different types of tissue. Adipose tissue is like marshmallow, oozy and fluffy. It takes up a lot of space. Muscle tissue, on the other hand, is dense and tight. It takes up very little space. Muscle, however, does not weigh more than adipose. What differs though is their density. Because muscle tissue is so dense, it takes up less space than adipose tissue making a person's appearance smaller or leaner.

The "Skinny-Fat Person"

Some obesity researchers now believe that the internal fat surrounding vital organs like the heart, liver, or pancreas, invisible to the naked eye, could be as dangerous as the more obvious external fat that bulges underneath the skin. In other words, being "thin" does not necessarily mean you are lean. A skinny-fat person, sometimes referred to as "thin outside, fat inside" (TOFI), typically has very little lean muscle mass and a lot of adipose tissue, which makes their total body weight appear normal.

In fact, fat, active people, sometimes called "fit and fat," can be healthier than their skinny, sedentary counterparts. Normal weight people who are sedentary and unfit are at much higher risk for developing disease than obese persons who are active and fit. How can this be?

Obesity researchers believe that people who are not overweight but still have a high percentage of body fat may have more inflammation in their bodies. These people are often referred to as "normal-weight obese" because of their high body fat percentage.

When researchers took blood samples from research subjects, they found those who were overweight or obese had the highest levels of inflammatory chemicals, LDL ("bad") cholesterol, and triglycerides (a type of blood fat). However, the "normal-weight obese" women also had higher levels of inflammatory chemicals than those with both a normal BMI and lower body fat. These findings indicate that the normal-weight women with high body fat "were in an early inflammatory state," because body fat is thought to release inflammatory chemicals, according to the researchers (De Lorenzo et al., 2007). Chronically high levels of inflammation have been associated with a host of health problems, including heart disease and arthritis.

Research also shows that people who maintain their weight through diet rather than exercise are likely to have major deposits of internal fat, even if they are otherwise slim. Typically, thin people may falsely assume that because they are not overweight, they are healthy.

In reality, a skinny fat person may have a "normal" weight, but this does not make them immune to diabetes or other risk factors for heart disease.

Skinny-fat people, who are fat on the inside, are essentially on the threshold of being obese. They eat too many fatty, sugary foods, and exercise too little to work it off, but they are not eating enough to actually be overweight.

Most experts believe that being of normal weight is an indicator of good health, and that BMI is a reliable measurement. BMI won't give you the exact indication of where fat is, but it can be a useful clinical tool. Still, getting a body composition assessment would be a better indicator of body fat percentage.

MEASURING BODY FAT PERCENTAGE

Two popular and often used techniques for measuring body fat include:

Skinfold Calipers

Skinfold calipers are a type of "old school" measurement that looks like kitchen tongs. They are used by "pinching" a fold of fat on different regions of the body such as the bicep, tricep, subscapular, above the hip bone, and sometimes on the calf. There is room for error, however, if the person performing the assessment "pinches" the skinfold too hard. This makes the person appear "leaner" than they really are. It's important that the technician (usually a personal trainer, dietician, or other health professional) measure the sites three separate times and then average his or her findings to account for human error.

Bio-electrical Impedance Analysis (BIA)

Bioelectrical impedance is measured when a very small electrical signal carried by water and fluids is passed through the body. Impedance is greatest in fat tissue (this interferes with the passing of the electrical current), which contains only 10 to 20 percent water, whereas fat-free mass, which contains 70 to 75 percent water, allows the signal to pass much more easily.

If a person is dehydrated, the amount of fat tissue can be overestimated. Factors that can affect hydration include not drinking enough fluids, drinking too much caffeine or alcohol, exercising or eating just before measuring, taking certain prescription drugs or diuretics, illness, or a woman's menstrual cycle. Measuring under consistent conditions is important to get accurate results with this method.

Tips to Improve Body Composition

- Commit to cardiovascular exercise at a vigorous intensity at least three days per week, preferably four or five. Interval training is great for reducing body fat and maintaining lean muscle tissue. Interval training is short bursts of intense cardiovascular exercise followed by rest and recovery periods of lower intensity work. For example, if you are on a treadmill, after warming up, you might sprint for 30 to 45 seconds and then recover by jogging or walking for 2 to 3 minutes. This cycle would then be repeated 4 to 5 times in a 30-minute session.

- Include weight training two to three times per week. Start with large muscle exercises that work areas such as the back, legs, arms, and chest. Start slowly, but work up to lifting a weight that is challenging. If you can easily lift a given weight 15 repetitions or more, consider increasing the weight. Remember, building muscle means making the body appear smaller and toned. Try weight training followed by a shorter cardio session. This offers the benefit of maximum strength for lifting and continued fat burning during the cardio.

- Eat protein with every meal, and try to eat every three hours. Protein is the building block of muscle, and it is essential for tissue repair.

- Round out your meals with complex carbohydrates like whole grains, fruits, vegetables, and legumes, and always eat within 45 minutes after exercise.

- Manage stress to reduce levels of the stress hormone cortisol, which can increase abdominal fat and muscle breakdown. Practice meditation, stretching, and/or yoga to help decrease stress levels.

CAUSES OF OBESITY

Many think of fat as greasy blobs stored under the skin, but it is now widely accepted that it behaves more like an active organ, constantly changing and sending out hormones that affect your mood, ability to think clearly, and fertility levels.

The fat just underneath the skin is called subcutaneous fat. Internal fat (the kind sitting around the abdomen and surrounding vital organs) is referred to as visceral fat.

Fat cells are kind of like "chemical factories" producing other substances and causing inflammation, which can cause long-term harm. They contribute to diabetes, heart disease, high blood pressure, strokes, and other illnesses, including some cancers.

If you eat more food calories than you burn, the excess is stored in your fat cells. How much fat a person has reflects both the number and the size of the fat cells (Whitney & Rolfes, 2002). During periods of rapid growth, such as puberty, fat cells increase significantly (Bray, 1992).

The only way to get rid of fat cells is through a cosmetic procedure, such as liposuction. In other words, fat cells can expand in size. And once they reach their maximum size, they may also divide. When you lose weight, the number of fat cells remains the same. They simply shrink in size, but do not go away.

As you put on more weight, the cells grow bigger, sending out messages to nearby cells, which start to divide to produce more fat cells. A lean adult has 40 billion fat cells; an obese adult has two to three times that.

Body shape is often governed by genetic factors. When both parents are overweight, their children have a high likelihood of also being overweight. People shaped like apples, carrying excess weight in the abdomen, are more at risk than those built like pears, who deposit fat in the hips, thighs, and backsides. Women tend to fall into the latter category. Constant dieting may interfere with the way the body lays down fat, and there is evidence that this will increase visceral fat.

Overeating is a major factor behind obesity. Food portion sizes have increased since the 1970s. Today, foods are king-sized, big-slam, and super-sized. With more Americans eating out and grabbing food on-the-go, it is no surprise that they are taking in more food calories than they need without realizing it.

For many people, eating is an action that occurs in response to psychological factors like boredom, anxiety, stress, anger, sadness, and happiness. When a person regularly eats for reasons other than biological hunger, that is, they are eating to satisfy their psychological appetite, they are likely to have a weight problem. Think about it. An animal in the wild will hunt its food and eat in response to the biological sign of hunger. It does not do this, however, because it had a bad day at work. Nor will it overeat. Once it is satisfied, the animal will cease eating.

Modern technology has replaced muscle activity at home and at work, which means we move less today than a century ago. Technology has contributed to a sedentary lifestyle among the American population. Picture the typical American's work day: They rise after sleeping (sedentary), sit down and eat breakfast (sedentary), and then get into their car to drive to work (sedentary). Once at work, they sit behind their desk in front of a computer (sedentary). Once the work day is finished, the person drives home (sedentary), eats dinner (sedentary), and relaxes in front of the television (sedentary) before going to bed (sedentary).

If you ask the average American whether or not they are sedentary, most will cry foul. However, they are confusing being *busy* with being *active*. Many Americans lead very hectic lives working, taking care of children and other family members, and going to school. All of these activities give the *perception* of a lifestyle that is anything but sedentary. Unless a person is elevating their heart rate through physical activity multiple times a week for a period of time, they are, in fact, sedentary.

The 3 Fat Hormones

1. **Insulin**—produced by the beta cells in the pancreas when there is a rise in blood glucose. Insulin is a storage hormone. Its function is to take nutrients from the bloodstream and store them in body cells. Since insulin is a storage hormone, it also stops the body from using fat as a fuel source.

   To keep insulin levels low:
   - Have many small meals throughout the day, because larger meals tend to cause a greater insulin response.
   - Watch your carbohydrate intake. Eating too many carbs in a meal increases the insulin response.
   - Eat more fiber and complex carbs and less simple carbs. So eat **more** broccoli, cauliflower, green beens, whole grains, squash, and yams and **less** bread, pasta, rice, cereals, and candy.

2. **Leptin**—primary function is to act on the hypothalamus, the part of the brain that signals satiety. It tells the hypothalamus to reduce appetite (because fat stores are high), which results in decreased food intake. When fat stores are low (after dieting or fasting or skipping meals), leptin levels are reduced and this causes the hypothalamus to increase appetite. Leptin is responsible for weight gain after a diet.

   Leptin resistance may also result from eating too much or binge eating. When someone over-eats, the receptors in the hypothalamus become de-sensitized to leptin. This means that the hypothalamus can't detect when leptin levels are high, resulting in food cravings and further weight gain.

   In order to prevent leptin resistance:
   - Do not diet and skip meals.
   - Do not overeat and consume too many calories.
   - Avoid excess sugar and bad fats.

- Exercise daily.
- Improve sleeping habits—poor sleeping habits cause leptin resistance because the sleep hormone, melatonin, appears to work closely with leptin.

3. **Ghrelin,** on the other hand, is a hormone produced mainly by cells lining the stomach and cells of the pancreas that stimulates appetite (Inui, 2004). Ghrelin levels increase before meals and decrease after meals. It is considered the counterpart of the hormone leptin. Ghrelin has a pleasure effect on the human sense and creates a happiness associated with food, similar to those who suffer from drug addictions. Lean people tend to produce more of this hormone than obese people. Therefore, have small, frequent meals throughout the day.

Disease States Associated with Overweight and Obesity

The bulk of diseases in the United States would be eradicated if obesity rates would normalize. The hard reality is that we are built to move. Exercise signals the body's cells to grow and be healthy instead of fading. The following are associated with being overweight or obese:

- Hypertension (high blood pressure)
- Osteoarthritis (a degeneration of cartilage and its underlying bone within a joint)
- Dyslipidemia (for example, high total cholesterol or high levels of triglycerides)
- Type 2 diabetes
- Coronary heart disease
- Stroke
- Gallbladder disease
- Sleep apnea and respiratory problems
- Some cancers (endometrial, breast, and colon)

Men who go from sedentary to fit cut their risk of heart disease by 75% over five years. For women, it's a whopping 80%. And don't forget, heart attacks are the largest single killer of women in the United States.

PHYSICAL ACTIVITY

As previously mentioned, people who combine diet with exercise tend to not only have lower rates of visceral fat, but also are more likely to maintain weight loss and have improved mood due to the psychological benefits of exercise. So, how much is enough?

It is generally acknowledged that you should work out at least three to five times per week. An exercise program should include both cardiovascular activities (e.g., running, stairclimbing, fast walking) and strength training.

Cardio should be done for 20 to 60 minutes. A person who has been sedentary should start slowly. Over time, stamina and cardiorespiratory function will increase, and the person will be able to go longer.

Strength training should be done 2 to 3 times per week with a focus on the major muscle groups: back, chest, thighs, gluteals, arms, and shoulders. A weight should be challenging enough that you cannot do any more than 15 repetitions. If you can do more than that using proper form, you should increase the weight that you are using.

The best place to start is simple: buy a pedometer. A pedometer is a step counter that you clip onto your belt loop. You should aim for 10,000 steps per day. Most Americans barely clear 2,500 steps a day! For most people, wearing a pedometer is a real wake-up call for just how sedentary they really are.

RESOURCES

Bray, G. A. 1992. Pathophysiology of obesity. *American Journal of Clinical Nutrition,* 55:488S–494S.

Centers For Disease Control and Prevention. U.S. Obesity Trends 1985–2007: *www.cdc.org*

De Lorenzo, A., et al. (2007). Normal-weight obese syndrome: early inflammation? *American Journal of Clinical Nutrition,* 85 (1):40–45.

Drummond, K. E. & Brefere, L. M. 2004. *Nutrition for foodservice and culinary professionals.* 5th ed. John Wiley & Sons, Inc.

Inui A., et al. 2004. Ghrelin, appetite, and gastric motility: the emerging role of the stomach as an endocrine organ. *Federation of American Societies for Experimental Biology Journal.* 18 (3): 439–56.

National Health and Nutrition Examination Survey (NHANES), 2003 to 2004. National Center for Health Statistics: *http://www.cdc.gov/nchs/about/major/nhanes/nhanes2003-2004/nhanes03_04.htm*

Roizen, M. F., Oz, M. C. 200. *You on a diet: The owner's manual for waist management.* Simon & Schuster, Inc.

U.S. Department of Health and Human Services. Healthy People 2010. 2nd ed. With Understanding and Improving Health and Objectives for Improving Health. 2 vols. Washington, DC: U.S. Government Printing Office, November 2000.

Wahrenberg, H. 2005. *British Medical Journal.* Online 1st ed., April 15.

Whitney, E. N., Rolfes, S. R. 2002. *Understanding Nutrition.* 9th ed. Wadsworth Thomson Learning.

chapter 9
Myths and Misconceptions

Fads abound in the field of nutrition and, naturally, so do a plethora of myths and misconceptions about what to eat, what not to eat, how to eat, and on and on. The growing relevance of nutrition and its relationship to disease prevention has piqued the interested of many "arm chair" nutritionists. That is, many lay people have become well-versed on basic nutrition principles. The problem, however, is that while they may have some things right, they often have many things wrong.

Many misperceptions exist within the field of nutrition and probably will only get worse as time goes on. The following "myths and misperceptions" have been compiled by the authors over many years of clinical practice and academic experience. Students continue to be a source of inspiration behind these "myths" often debunking them on their own once they've taken this class! We encourage all of you to practice becoming a critical consumer, read food labels and nutritional claims carefully and soon you'll be able to food shop and eat with confidence!

MYTHS AND MISPERCEPTIONS

*In no particular order

Sugar Causes Diabetes

Hands down, when teaching about diabetes, this myth is a repeat offender. It seems that people have interpreted the notion that too much sugar in the blood is what causes diabetes, when in, fact, elevated blood sugar is really the *symptom* of a greater underlying problem. Let's review what's going on when a person has diabetes. First some definitions:

Hormone: A chemical "messenger." Delivers a product from point A to point B.
Insulin: Hormone responsible for delivering glucose from point A: the blood stream, to Point B: the body's cells.
Pancreas: Endocrine organ responsible for secreting the hormone insulin.

There are two main types of diabetes: Type 1 and Type 2.

Type 1 is an autoimmune disease. In other words, your lifestyle behaviors did not contribute to the onset of your illness. Typically people diagnosed with Type 1 diabetes are under 25 years old. This type used to be referred to as juvenile-onset. With this type of diabetes, certain cells of the pancreas responsible for making insulin are not working. Insulin must be injected daily for life.

Type 2 diabetes is the result of lifestyle behaviors such as being overweight or obese, as well as being sedentary. Old age can also be a cause of Type 2 diabetes. In very rare cases, trauma or injury to the body can also contribute to the onset of type 2 diabetes.

With this type of diabetes, the pancreas does work and is manufacturing insulin. However, the body's cells are "resistant" to it because of overweight/obesity/sedentary lifestyle, etc.

When we eat foods that contain carbohydrates (grains, fruits, veggies, legumes, nuts), there is a normal rise in blood sugar levels (glucose). Insulin comes along (once the pancreas is alerted to the rise in blood sugar) and carries some of the sugar from the meal or snack in the bloodstream to the body's cells where it can be used as energy. In a person with type 1 diabetes, they would have to inject the necessary insulin. In a person with type 2 diabetes, the insulin is secreted and carries the sugar (from the bloodstream) to the body's cells, but the cells will not accept the sugar. They are *resistant* to the insulin. In other words, the cells don't respond to the insulin. As a result, the sugar has nowhere to go (can't enter the cells like it's supposed to) and blood sugar stays elevated. This elevation in blood sugar sends *another* signal to the pancreas to crank out even more insulin, so the whole process can be attempted once more. Again, the same result happens: the cells are insulin resistant. Eventually, the pancreas grows tired of sending out insulin and sputters out. Only through proper diet and vigorous exercise will the cells become responsive to insulin again.

So, if you have diabetes, you do need to watch your sugar and carbohydrate intake to properly manage your blood sugar levels. However, if you do not have diabetes, sugar intake will not cause you to develop the disease. The main risk factors for type 2 diabetes are a diet high in calories, being overweight, and a sedentary lifestyle.

Eating Fat is Bad Especially if You Want to Lose Weight

One myth that just won't go away is that if you eat fat, you'll be fat.

It's a long-held nutrition myth that all fats are bad. But the fact is, we all need fat. Let's recap what fat does:

- Cushions organs
- Acts as an insulator (helps regulate body temperature)
- Helps transport fat-soluble vitamins: A, D, E, K
- Aids nerve transmission
- Helps maintain cell membrane integrity
- Helps promote satiety—keeps you feeling satisfied longer in between meals so you're less likely to snack mindlessly.

Not all fats are created equal. Some fats can actually help promote good health, while others can clog blood vessels and inflammation. It's important to remember that all fats contain 9 calories per gram consumed. They are very energy dense. The general rule of thumb for fats is this: Saturated fats are typically solid at room temperature and come from the animal kingdom with the exception of tropical oils. Unsaturated fats are typically liquid at room temperature and come from the plant kingdom with the exception of seafood like fish. Let's recap our fats:

Unsaturated fats are healthy:
- Olive oil
- Canola oil
- Fatty fish like sardines, halibut, salmon, bluefish, mackerel
- Flaxseed
- Nuts like walnuts
- Soy found in tofu
- Avocado

Saturated fats are unhealthy:

- Lard
- Butter
- Tropical oils like coconut oil, cocoa butter, palm oil
- Marbling on cuts of beef, pork, lamb
- Skin on poultry
- Processed foods like cookies, cakes, candies, and chips

Trans fats:

- Processed foods like cookies, cakes, crackers, candy, cereals, breads
- Look for the words "partially hydrogenated." If you see these words, it indicates that trans fats are present in the food product.

Remember, if you eat more food calories than your body needs, you store them as body fat. It doesn't matter where those calories come from (fat or carbohydrate or protein). If you eat more than you need, you store it as fat.

Carbohydrates are "Fattening"

This is inherently false since you now know that carbohydrate-rich foods contain little, if any, lipid. It's not until we *add* a lipid that they become fattening: cream cheese or butter to your bagel, alfredo sauce or pesto to your pasta, sour cream and cheese to your potato.

When people go on a low carbohydrate diet they often do lose weight. But not for the reasons you think. Many low carbohydrate diets actually do not provide sufficient carbohydrates to your body for daily maintenance. Therefore your body will begin to burn stored carbohydrates (glycogen) for energy. When your body starts burning glycogen, water is released. In fact, for every gram of carbohydrate, a molecule of water is attached to it. That drastic initial drop of weight at the beginning of a low carbohydrate diet is mostly the water that you lose as a result of burning glycogen. So, you've lost water weight, NOT body fat.

The fact is, to lose body fat, you must take in fewer calories than your body needs, plus exercise. A low carbohydrate diet gives the perception that you're eating a lot. This is because you're usually eating "forbidden" foods like butter, mayonnaise, fatty meats, creamy salad dressings, and cheese. In reality, low carbohydrate diets tend to be lower in calories than traditional diets, thus the weight loss. Here's an example.

Let's say today you are NOT on a low carbohydrate diet. You and a friend decide to eat out at a steakhouse. Your dinner begins with bread from the breadbasket. Next, an appetizer followed by the entrée of a steak, loaded baked potato, and a vegetable side. For dessert, a slice of carrot cake. All of this is washed down by a glass of red wine.

Now, let's say that tomorrow I AM on a low carbohydrate diet. Look at the above meal. What exactly will I be eating? Bread? No. Appetizer? Maybe. Steak? Yes. Potato? No. Veggie side? Maybe. Carrot cake? No. Red wine? No.

So, which meal has fewer calories—the low carbohydrate day or the "normal" day? Explain

_____

_____

_____

_____

_____

_____

_____

You're correct if you said the low carbohydrate day.

The problem with avoiding carbohydrates long-term is that it becomes very difficult to maintain. So while you initially lose weight, many people regain the weight and more once they start eating carbohydrates again.

Brown Sugar is Healthier than White Sugar

Students consistently believe this myth. The fact is, however, sugar is sugar is sugar is sugar! It doesn't matter whether you eat white sugar or brown sugar or raw sugar, to your body it's all the same thing. And chemically, it is. It is all made of:

Fructose + Glucose

In fact, the brown sugar sold at grocery stores is actually white granulated sugar with added molasses.

The main reason that there are so many different types of sugar is strictly for baking purposes. Brown sugar, for example, has a high moisture content and, therefore, will make quick breads and cakes more moist. But at the end of the day, there is no health benefit to selecting one sugar over another. A baking benefit, yes. A health benefit, no.

The one exception to the "sugar is sugar is sugar is sugar" rule is something called high fructose corn syrup. The following is an excerpt from the *San Francisco Chronicle*. Nationally recognized nutrition expert Mario Nestle answers readers' questions in a column entitled, Food Matters. This Q & A is specifically about high fructose corn syrup (September 24, 2008).

_____

Q: What is the difference, metabolically speaking, between high-fructose corn syrup and other carbohydrate-based sweeteners (sucrose, fructose, honey, and so on)?

A: From what I hear these days, high-fructose corn syrup (HFCS) is widely perceived as the new trans fat, something to be avoided at all costs. But, stop: HFCS is not poison. It is just sugar in liquid form, differing from common table sugar (sucrose) mainly in how it affects the texture of foods.

I can see why HFCS seems like a nutritional villain: It is a marker for junk foods. Cheaper than sucrose, it turns up in all kinds of processed foods, particularly soft drinks. And there is nearly as much of it in the food supply as sucrose—56 pounds per year per person versus 62 pounds for table sugar.

In its new advertising campaign, the Corn Refiners Association says of HFCS, "Truth is, it's nutritionally the same as table sugar." Truth is, I'd call it almost the same.

Sucrose is a double sugar made of two single sugars—glucose (50 percent) and fructose (50 percent)—stuck together. HFCS also contains glucose and fructose, but the sugars are already separated and their percentages differ slightly. Because sucrose is quickly split by digestive enzymes, the body can hardly tell them apart. For the record, glucose is blood sugar, fructose is fruit sugar, and honey contains both.

The processing of sucrose involves boiling it down from sugar cane or beets, and washing, clarifying, filtering and drying the syrup. HFCS starts out as corn, of course, and you, too, can do what the makers of the indie movie, "King Corn" (2007), demonstrated in my favorite scene.

First, extract the starch. Use enzymes to break down the starch to glucose and to convert some of the glucose to fructose. Then do a bunch of refining, separation and evaporation steps. The resulting syrup is 55 percent fructose, with the rest composed of glucose or undigested starch pieces. The HFCS used in soft drinks has a bit more fructose than sucrose—55 percent as opposed to 50 percent.

Whether this 5 percent difference matters at all depends on whether you are a metabolic optimist or pessimist.

If you are an optimist, you are happy that fructose—unlike glucose—does not stimulate the release of insulin, and in small amounts can be a useful sweetener for people with diabetes.

If you are a pessimist, you will fret that fructose is preferentially metabolized to fat, raising the possibility that HFCS—or any other source of fructose (but we won't worry about fruit)—could have something to do with current obesity trends.

HFCS entered our food supply in the mid 1960s, but did not really come into its own until farm subsidies encouraged farmers to grow as much corn as possible. In 1981, at the dawn of the obesity era, the United States food supply provided 23 pounds of HFCS per person per year, along with 79 pounds of sucrose—102 pounds total.

Today, the balance is 56 to 62 (118 pounds), with the increase entirely due to HFCS. Guilt by association! Glucose corn syrups and honey add up to yet another 18 pounds, but their use has not changed much over time. All told, the food supply provides a third of a pound a day of HFCS and sucrose combined, which works out to about 600 calories a day per person, just from these two sources.

Note that these are available calories, not necessarily those eaten. Availability refers to sugars produced, plus imports, less exports. Even so, people who drink sodas all day long can get a substantial portion of their daily calories from HFCS. Like other sugars, HFCS supplies calories but is devoid of nutrients.

Although only about 6 percent of U.S. corn is used to make corn sweeteners, it is 6 percent of a large number. Corn production is subsidized, and subsidies encourage greater production. Until recently, subsidies drove the cost of corn sweeteners well below that of sucrose, which gets price supports. With corn now going for ethanol, HFCS is more expensive and has less of a price advantage.

Indeed, some food companies have already replaced HFCS with sucrose and are advertising their products as "HFCS-free." At least one grocery chain has said it will no longer carry products containing HFCS. Such events, along with concerns about the metabolic effects of fructose, saddle the Corn Refiners with a challenge—how to convince the American public that HFCS is no worse than any other sugar.

Their methods? First, they successfully petitioned the Food and Drug Administration to allow HFCS to be labeled "natural." Despite the many steps required to process cornstarch into HFCS, the FDA granted their request. Why? Because in processing the enzymes are fixed to a column and the sugars do not come in contact with the synthetic fixing agents. I'm not kidding about this.

Next, the Corn Refiners funded a $30 million counterattack. If you missed the full-page newspaper ads, take a look at the web site, www.sweetsurprise.com.

HFCS has a big public relations problem, but I don't get this campaign. Since when is insulting the intelligence of critics an effective marketing strategy?

I cannot decide which aspects of the campaign are most offensive: The videos of inarticulate critics insulted by their HFCS-savvy friends? The slogans ("HFCS has no artificial ingredients")? The quiz questions ("Which of the following sweeteners is considered a natural food ingredient:

HFCS, honey, sugar, or all of the above")? Or the irrelevant take-home message ("As registered dietitians recommend, keep enjoying the foods you love, just do it in moderation")?

I'm not a registered dietitian and maybe that is why I think moderation doesn't work for HFCS. Yes, HFCS has a place in the American diet and sometimes has cooking advantages over sucrose. And the research is still out on whether HFCS differs from sucrose metabolically. But the most sensible approach to HFCS and to sugars in general is not moderation. It is, "Eat less."

Eating Eggs or Shrimp Raise Blood Cholesterol

There is a growing body of evidence demonstrating that the majority of people will have relatively small cholesterol changes in response to changes in dietary cholesterol intake. In other words, eating dietary cholesterol (particularly rich in eggs and shrimp) has less of an effect on cholesterol levels than consuming foods high in saturated and *trans* fats. What becomes essential for effective interventions to lower cholesterol levels is an overall lowering of saturated and trans fat intake and an increase in vigorous physical activity most days of the week. The majority of data available shows that the addition of eggs (at two per day) to the diet of healthy people has little effect on plasma cholesterol levels (Ginsberg et al., 1995; Ferrier et al. 1995; Knopp et al. 1996)

The same is true for shrimp and other seafood. Dietary cholesterol found in shrimp and other seafood has little effect on blood cholesterol in most people. Saturated fats and *trans* fatty acids are the most important factors that raise blood cholesterol.

Keep in mind, too, that when many people consume shrimp or other seafood, it's often fried in an unhealthy fat or "dipped" in butter. Implementing a healthy cooking technique is vital to ensuring a lower intake of saturated fat, which is a contributor to elevated blood cholesterol.

Don't Eat Nuts—Too Fattening!

It is true that nuts are very high in fat and, therefore, quite high in calories. One ounce of walnuts, for example, which is about a small handful, contains 183 calories (USDA's National Nutrient Database for Standard Reference). The key with eating nuts is to do so in moderation. They are very easy to overeat and, as a result, take in a lot of extra calories. Still, nuts can be a part of a healthy diet. In fact, as previously discussed, nuts are high in monounsaturated and polyunsaturated fats (the good fats) as well as plant sterols, all of which have been shown to lower LDL cholesterol.

In 2003, the FDA approved a health claim for seven kinds of nuts stating that "scientific evidence suggests but does not prove that eating 1.5 ounces (45 grams) per day of most nuts as part of a diet low in saturated fat and cholesterol may reduce the risk of heart disease." Instead of simply adding nuts to your diet, the best approach is to eat them in replacement of foods high in saturated fats.

Eat 2–3 Meals If You Want to Lose Weight

People who skip meals, especially breakfast, tend to get so hungry that they overeat their next meal or snack to compensate for feeling so hungry. This starts a vicious cycle of binge eating and restricting that is not only mentally exhausting, but counterproductive to long-term fat loss. When you skip meals, your metabolism (the rate at which you burn calories) tends to slow down. Eating small meals and snacks (say, three moderate meals and two small snacks) throughout the day helps people control their appetites and their weight!

Don't Eat After 8 PM if You Want to Lose Weight

Have you ever been to Spain or France or another European country? If so, you probably noticed that they tend to eat their dinner meal very late compared to the typical American. And, yet, they stay slim. What's going on here?

First, each of us is allotted a certain number of calories to be consumed in a 24-hour time span. Your body does not care when those calories are consumed. Let's say you're driving down the highway at two in the morning and you notice that your car's gas meter is on "E," for empty. You're not going to say, "I can't fill up my gas tank because it's after 8 PM," are you? Of course not.

The problem with most Americans is not eating after 8 PM. It's that most *overeat* after 8 PM. See the difference?

Here's the typical American eating profile:

- 6:00 AM—out of bed, off to work/school, no breakfast consumed
- 7–8 AM—grab coffee on the go
- 10 AM—maybe another coffee
- 12 PM—small salad, diet coke for lunch
- 4 PM—gummy bears, diet coke from vending machine.
- 6 PM—General Tso's chicken and rice from Chinese restaurant
- 8 PM—watch television and snack on a bag of chips
- 11 PM—2 bowls of ice cream while watching nightly news
- 12 AM—finish off leftover General Tso's chicken and rice and wash it down with some soda before bed

When the person wakes up 5–6 hours later, they're not hungry for breakfast, so it's skipped (again). But, why would they be after eating so much not so long ago? And then the cycle starts all over again for another day.

It does not matter what time of day you eat. It is what and how much you eat as well as how much physical activity you do during a 24-hour time span that determines whether you gain, lose, or maintain weight. No matter when you eat, if you do not use all the calories that you have consumed, your body will store the extra calories as fat. Keep in mind, though: It is a good idea to consume the bulk of your calories during the time of day that you are most active.

I'm Skinny, So I Can Eat Whatever I Want

Recall the previous discussion of the "skinny-fat person." We now know that being "skinny" or "thin" doesn't guarantee that you are lean. A skinny-fat person, sometimes referred to as "thin outside, fat inside" (TOFI), typically has very little lean muscle mass and a lot of adipose tissue which makes their total body weight appear normal.

In fact, fat, active people, sometimes called "fit and fat," can be healthier than their skinny, sedentary counterparts. Normal weight people who are sedentary and unfit are at much higher risk for developing disease than obese persons who are active and fit. How can this be?

Obesity researchers believe that people who aren't overweight but still have a high percentage of body fat may have more inflammation in their bodies. These people are often referred to as "normal-weight obese" because of their high body fat percentage.

Chronically high levels of inflammation have been associated with a host of health problems, including heart disease, stroke, hypertension, and arthritis.

In reality, a skinny-fat person may have a "normal" weight, but this doesn't make them immune to diabetes or other risk factors for heart disease.

If you are trying to maintain or even lose weight, a healthy diet and exercise can help you increase your lean tissue (muscle) while decreasing your fat stores. This will help increase your metabolism which will help you burn calories at a quicker rate. Regular physical activity and a healthy diet can help you strengthen your lungs and blood vessels, which can prevent or prolong heart disease. Physical activity and a healthy diet can also improve your blood cholesterol level.

I'm Pregnant, So I'm 'Eating for Two'

You learn you're pregnant and you immediately think, "Bring on the pizza and ice cream!" Unfortunately, the idea that pregnancy is an ice cream free-for-all is a nutrition myth. It is generally recommended that pregnant women increase their daily intake by 100 calories in the first trimester, which is less than one can of Coke! During the second and third trimesters, 300 extra calories per day is recommended.

Being pregnant is not a license to consume whatever you want. The quality of calories consumed is important to ensure the mother's health and the baby's growth and development. Moms-to-be should choose nutrient-rich foods like whole grains, low-fat dairy products, legumes, and fruits and vegetables, which are high in essential nutrients compared to their calorie count.

A daily prenatal multivitamin supplement is often recommended during pregnancy, but you should always talk with your doctor before taking any vitamin/mineral supplements.

Coffee Can Help You Lose Weight

While coffee and other caffeine products like soda, tea, and Red Bull may temporarily squelch your appetite, drinking a couple of cups a day won't have enough of an effect to help you lose weight. Drinking four to seven cups a day may lead to anxiety, sleeplessness, and an increase in heart rate and blood pressure.

Enjoy a cup or two of coffee every day, but remember that anything added like cream, sugar, or syrup will also add calories. For example, a 16-ounce Starbucks café mocha can contain a whopping 330 calories (60 more than some chocolate bars).

Another caffeine concern: sleep disruption, which new evidence reveals is linked to weight control. People become addicted to caffeine especially when sleep-deprived and it takes four to six hours to clear out of the system. Drinking caffeine is a quick fix because it only energizes you for 20–40 minutes and then you crash. After you crash, your body craves more caffeine or sugar to boost the energy and now you are setting the stage for a sugar/caffeine roller coaster which increases your appetite and promotes fat storage. At least two studies have shown that when people are sleep-deprived, they produce more of the hormone ghrelin, an appetite stimulant, and less leptin, an appetite suppressant.

Going on a Diet is the Best Way to Lose Weight

The first 3 letters of the word diet (**die**) should give you an indication of how **diets** fail and make you feel miserable.

Short-term, you do lose weight on any plan that results in your eating fewer calories. But temporary changes don't lead to permanent losses.

Sure, if you subsist on less than 1,200 calories a day, you'll take off weight, but it won't be for long. Consider an analysis of 31 studies of long-term diets, where the diets averaged 1,200 calories a day. The report, published last April in *American Psychologist,* found that within four to five years, the majority of dieters in these studies regained the weight they had lost. Psychologically, it's difficult for people to adhere to strict diets over a long period because they feel deprived and hungry. In addition, people who are put on a very low-calorie diet (800 calories a day) have an increased risk of developing gallstones and digestive issues and their metabolism slows down which will impair future weight loss.

Don't go on a "diet" which is usually just a quick fix that begins on New Year's Day. Instead, change the way you eat. Find a satisfying eating plan that you can live with long-term, and make sure you're eating the right amount of calories for weight loss.

But what's the right number of calories for you? Use this easy formula, a favorite of cardiologist Thomas Lee, editor in chief of the *Harvard Heart Letter*.

First, find your activity level on the table below. Multiply your weight by the number indicated. (You may fall between two categories. If that's the case, adjust the number by adding a point or so.) The result is the number of calories you need to maintain your weight. Let's say you weigh 135 pounds and do light exercise one to three days a week. Multiply 135 by 13.5 to get, approximately, 1,800 calories. If you want to drop some pounds, try cutting out 250 calories a day. In a year, if you make no other changes, you could be 26 pounds lighter.

If . . .

You Exercise: Almost never
Multiply Your Current Weight By: 12

You Exercise: Lightly, one to three days a week
Multiply Your Current Weight By: 13.5

You Exercise: Moderately, three to five days a week
Multiply Your Current Weight By: 15.5

You Exercise: Vigorously, six to seven days a week
Multiply Your Current Weight By: 17

You Exercise: Vigorously, daily, and you have a physical job
Multiply Your Current Weight By: 19

One of the most important aspects of weight maintenance is a high dose of physical activity. The National Weight Control Registry has followed and analyzed the habits of successful weight losers (defined as people who have maintained at least a 30-pound weight loss for a year or more). Among its findings: Those who kept weight off exercised—with brisk walking or some other moderate-intensity activity—an average of one hour a day.

Remember that 1 lb of fat = 3500 calories

So if you want to lose 1 lb of fat/week, eat 500 calories LESS per day
or burn an extra 500 calories from exercise or better yet, do both

---

Eating Protein and Carbohydrates at Different Meals Will Help You Lose Weight.

Your digestive tract can handle a variety of food groups at the same time. There is no proof that eating protein and carbohydrates separately aids digestion or weight loss. Most dietitians agree that it's healthier to combine protein and fiber-filled carbs than to separate them. The pairing of protein and fiber is what fills you up the most and gives you the most energy. An apple is good, but an apple with peanut butter is more filling and controls your blood sugar better.

Eat protein along with carbs, but choose those that are lower in fat. The best protein choices are lean meats, poultry, low-fat dairy products, and tofu. The best carbs are whole grains, fruits, and vegetables. These foods combined take longer to absorb, so there's a slower release into the body and a more steady energy source.

NUTRITION ASSIGNMENT # 9

1. Quiz a family member or friend on some of the nutrition myths from this chapter. Describe which ones they got wrong and why they believe those myths. Be sure to explain the correct answer to those that they got incorrect!

_____

_____

_____

_____

_____

_____

_____

_____

_____

_____

_____

2. Which myths from this chapter were you most surprised to learn? Describe below how you will do things differently in the future related to that myth.

_____

_____

_____

_____

_____

_____

_____

_____

_____

_____

_____

_____

3. Do you think you follow a nutritional myth? What is it and where did you learn about it?

_____

_____

_____

_____

_____

_____

_____

_____

_____

_____

_____

_____

_____

_____

_____

REFERENCES

Ferrier et al. 1995. Alpha-linolenic acid- and docosahexanaenoic acid-enriched eggs from hens fed flaxseed: influence on blood lipids and platelet phospholipid fatty acids in humans. Am. J. Clin. Nutr. 62:81–86.

Ginsberg et al. 1995. Increases in dietary cholesterol are associated with modest increases in both LDL and HDL cholesterol in healthy young women. Arterioscler. Thromb. Vasc. Biol. 15:169–178.

Knopp et al. 1996. A double-blind, randomized trial of the effects of two eggs per day in moderately hypercholesterolemic and combined hyperlipidemic subjects consuming the NCEP Step I diet. (Reported in abstract at the November 1995 American Heart Association meeting in Anaheim, CA).

Nestle, Marion. September 24, 2008: The Facts About Corn Sweetener. The *San Francisco Chronicle*: *http://sfgate.com/cgi-bin/article.cgi?f=/c/a/2008/09/24/FDDS12UH12.DTL* This article appeared on page F–1.

United States Department of Agriculture (USDA): *www.usda.gov*

chapter 10
Eating Better in America: Putting It All Together!

WHAT EATING HEALTHIER WILL DO FOR YOU

Eating healthy food will help you to:

- Feel great and have energy to enjoy life more
- Have a strong immune system so you stay well, even when everyone else is getting sick
- Maintain a healthy weight and look physically fit
- Stay as alert and mentally sharp at 60, 70, and even 80 as you were at 20
- Do the same things at 65 that you did at 20, with the same gusto
- Live to be 100, and be physically fit and active
- Prevent certain diseases known to be related to diet and nutrition, particularly cancer, heart disease, stroke, high blood pressure, high cholesterol, diabetes, and obesity

Some of the things that you could experience if you are not eating healthfully might include:

- Headaches
- Indigestion
- Depression
- Candida yeast
- Difficulty sleeping
- Poor memory
- Senile dementia
- Anorexia and bulimia
- Dry skin
- Adult acne
- Constipation
- Poor digestion
- Halitosis (bad breath)
- Mouth and tongue ulcers
- Menstrual problems
- Diarrhea
- Irritability
- Fatigue
- Polyps
- Diverticulitis

- Gallstones
- Osteoporosis
- COPD—(chronic obstructive pulmonary disease)
- Anemia
- Asthma
- Mental illness
- Irritable bowel syndrome
- Fibromyalgia

Our fast-food culture is one where meals have become yet another task that we squeeze in during the day. American adults devote an average of 1 hour and 12 minutes per day to eating, yet spend between 2 and 3 hours per day watching television. American youth kids are rushed, too. Studies have shown that school lunch periods provide an average of 7 to 11 minutes for students to consume their lunch.

Healthy eating is not about strict dieting, staying unrealistically thin, or depriving yourself of the foods you love; instead it is about feeling great, having more energy, and keeping yourself as healthy as possible.

When you want to lose weight, is your first choice to run to the latest fad diet? Often a quick 5 to 10 pounds will come off, then your old eating habits return and you end up gaining more weight and slowing down your metabolism. Preoccupation with body shape, size, and weight creates an unhealthy lifestyle of emotional and physical deprivation.

Decades of research have shown that diets, both self-initiated and professionally led, are ineffective at producing long-term health and weight loss or weight control. Only 5 percent of people who go on diets are successful; 95 percent of all traditional diets fail. When you go on a low-calorie diet, your body thinks you are starving. It actually becomes more efficient at storing fat by slowing down your metabolism. When you stop dieting, your metabolism is still slow and inefficient and you gain the weight back even faster. In addition, low-calorie diets cause you to lose both muscle and fat in equal amounts. However, when you eventually gain back the weight, it is all fat and not muscle, causing your metabolism to slow down even more.

Staying healthy is a life-long proposition. Do not waste your time, energy, and money on "quick fix" solutions. Fad diets, diet pills, protein powders, liposuction, and even intestinal or gastric bypass surgery might provide a leaner profile, but they do not provide the nutrients needed to keep you as healthy as you could be.

You should also consider that most diets are a temporary fix and may not result in your goal of long-term weight loss. As you consider each of these diets, note the number of calories it allows.

Comparison of Calories Among Major Diet Books

Book	Calories	Calorie Source	Claims	Points to Consider
Eat More, Weigh Less by Dean Ornish, MD	1,500	80% carbohydrates (CHO), 15% proteins, 5% fat, 40 g fiber	Fat free is key to weight loss.	Without a dietician's help, hard to maintain with so little fat. Fat provides flavor and texture to our food.

(continued)

Comparison of Calories Among Major Diet Books (Continued)

Book	Calories	Calorie Source	Claims	Points to Consider
Sugar Busters by Steward, Andrews, and Balart	1,600	35% CHO, 25% proteins, 40% fat, 20 g fiber	Refined CHO cause weight gain by raising blood sugar.	There is no scientific evidence to support this claim.
Dr. Atkins' Diet Revolution by Robert Atkins, MD	1,800	15% CHO, 30% proteins, 55% fat, 10g fiber	Only CHO make you fat. Eliminate them and your body burns fat.	There is no scientific evidence to support this claim. If you eliminate some calories, no matter what the source, your body must find energy elsewhere.
Protein Power by Michael and Mary Dan Eades	1,700	15% CHO, 25% proteins, 60% fat, 50 g fiber	Limits CHO; lowers insulin and insulin causes obesity.	This claim has been refuted by scientific research. It would be hard to maintain on this diet because CHOs are ubiquitous. We also know that a diet with 60% fat will increase your risk for heart disease. The diet does not allow for individual variation.
The Zone by Barry Sears	1,000	40% CHO, 30% proteins, 30% fat, 50 g fiber	Claims the FDA 60:15:30 ratio of CHO, protein, and fats causes weight gain. Changing to his 40:30:30 plan will result in weight loss.	The ratio is not the problem; the number of calories is the problem!
Dieting with the Duchess by Weight Watchers	1,400	55% CHO, 25% proteins, 20% fats, 25 g fiber	Food choices based on point system. Eat only the required points, you lose weight.	An easy to maintain calorie reduction method, with appropriate choices. This has been shown to produce long-term success.
The South Beach Diet by Arthur Agatston, MD	No calorie count is specified, but calories are greatly reduced in the first 2 weeks by eliminating CHO and fruit.	Emphasizes healthy fats, and allows only low glycemic index CHO. No bread, potatoes, fruits, corn, carrots, rice, or cereal in first 2 weeks and strongly discouraged even after the initiation phase.	Claims foods that are high on the glycemic index result in more weight gain.	The diet restricts many healthful food choices. There is no science to support that these high glycemic index foods lead to more weight gain. Exercise is not promoted.

Healthy eating is not just what you eat, but how you eat. Paying attention to what you eat and choosing foods that are both nourishing and enjoyable helps support an overall healthy diet. A better plan for healthy eating is one that is comprised of nutrient dense calories from all the essential food groups together with an exercise plan to which you can adhere. However, even this new healthy eating plan will not work unless you become responsible for what you eat, responsible for exercising, and accountable when you relapse. If you do relapse, just remember the days when you were successful and get back on track.

- Take time to chew your food. Chew your food slowly, savoring every bite. We tend to rush though our meals, forgetting to actually taste the flavors and feel the textures of what is in our mouths.
- Avoid eating while stress. When we are stressed, our digestion can be compromised, causing problems like colitis and heartburn. Avoid eating while working, driving, arguing, or watching television. Try taking some deep breaths before beginning your meal.
- Stop multi-tasking. We often pair eating with other activities, such as driving or working at our desks. Eating while multitasking, whether working through lunch or watching television while eating dinner, often leads us to eat more.
- Listen to your body. Ask yourself if you are really hungry, and stop eating when you feel full. It actually takes a few minutes for your brain to tell your body that it has had enough food, so eat slowly.
- Eat mindfully. Eating mindfully means eating with awareness—not awareness of what foods are on your plate, but rather awareness of the experience of eating. Mindful eating is being present, moment by moment, for each sensation that happens during eating, such as chewing, tasting and swallowing. Mindless eating, or eating without awareness, can have negative health consequences. It turns out that when our mind is tuned out during mealtime, the digestive process may be 30 percent to 40 percent less effective, which can contribute to digestive distress, such as gas, bloating, and bowel irregularities, overeating, and obesity.

HOW TO PRACTICE EATING MINDFULLY

Mindful eating means paying attention to what you eat and savoring each bite. Being mindful also means noticing when you are almost full and laying down your fork. Mindful eating relaxes you so you digest better and makes you feel more satisfied.

Eat with awareness of the taste, chew, bite, or swallow. Try the following exercise.

1. Take one bite of an apple slice (or any food) and then close your eyes. Do not begin chewing yet.
2. Try not to pay attention to the ideas running through your mind, just focus on the apple. Notice anything that comes to mind about taste, texture, temperature, and sensation going on in your mouth.
3. Begin chewing now. Chew slowly, just noticing what it feels like. It is normal that your mind will want to wander off. If you notice that you are paying more attention to your thinking than to the chewing, just let go of the thought for the moment and come back to the chewing. Notice each tiny movement of your jaw.
4. In these moments, you may find yourself wanting to swallow the apple. See if you can stay present and notice the subtle transition from chewing to swallowing.

5. As you prepare to swallow the apple, try to follow it moving toward the back of your tongue and into your throat. Swallow the apple, following it until you can no longer feel any sensation of the food remaining.

6. Take a deep breath and exhale.

DIET STRATEGIES THAT WORK

- Choose foods that contain fewer calories and more fiber, which will fill you up.
- Eating five smaller meals might work better than eating three larger ones. The goal is to eat a small amount of food every three hours or so.
- Eat less cholesterol and less fat, especially less saturated fat and no trans fat. Fats are very high in calories.
- Eat more fiber to fool your stomach. Reduce the calories by focusing on water-dense fruits and vegetables; therefore, you can keep the volume high and feel satisfied. Your stomach senses food volume, it has stretch receptors and pressure sensors. Start meals with a big salad—lots of vegetables with no croutons or creamy dressing like Caesar dressing; have double portions of fruit and vegetables at meals and skip or cut back on calorie-dense starches, fats, and fatty meats. Opt for a fruit dessert, with a dab of sorbet for flavor.
- Eat quality carbohydrates. Choosing low glycemic foods like fruits, vegetables, and whole grains over refined foods (e.g., sodas, doughnuts, white potatoes) could help keep you from gaining ten extra pounds even if you do not cut calories. Low-glycemic eating makes blood sugar stay lower, you feel full faster, and the body does not seem to react to the diet with as much stress.
- Choose whole grain cereal, pasta, rice, and bread. Many foods that claim they are "whole wheat" or "whole grain" on the front of the package are really made with mostly white processed flour, which is not nearly as nutritious. Always check the ingredients to see if "whole wheat" or "whole grain" is the first ingredient listed; do not be fooled by how a food looks. For example, some dark brown breads are colored with coffee or other dyes, not whole grains.
- Avoid food that is high in sugar, like pastries, sweetened cereal, and soda or fruit-flavored drinks.
- Watch what you drink.

Beverage	Calories/16 Ounces
Ice cream milk shakes	538
Grape juice	307
Orange juice	224
Cola	200
Iced teas, sugared	200
Beer	195
Sports drinks	100
Water	0

- Reduced-fat or no-fat (skim) milk, reduced-fat cheese, and low-fat or no-fat yogurt are good sources of needed protein and calcium.
- Exercise more to burn calories. Research has shown that 30 minutes of moderately strenuous daily exercise is also one of the most important requirements for disease prevention—even for people who are already at an ideal weight. For example 3,400 more steps a day for 3 months will do the following for you:

  3.3 pounds lost
  0.6-point reduction in BMI
  1-centimeter drop in waist circumference
  4-beat-per-minute drop in resting heart rate
  11,550 extra calories burned

- Eat nuts. The protein, fat, and fiber in almonds keep you feeling full. Have a handful (no more they are also high in calories) in place of your usual midmorning or afternoon snack.
- Let the sun in. A host of solid new studies from leading institutions link light deprivation to a wide variety of weight-related disorders including depression, bulimia, and PMS. People who are chronically deprived of light exposure can have profound effects on dietary choices, energy levels, physical activity, and weight gain. Susceptible people experience overwhelming food cravings, lethargy, and weight gain (some more than 30 pounds) during dark winter months.
- Get a good night's sleep. Lack of sleep may pack on extra pounds. In a recent study at the University of Chicago, people who slept only four hours a night for two nights had a 28% higher level of ghrelin (the eat-more hormone) and an 18% lower level of leptin (the eat-less hormone) than those who slept more (Ann of Int Med, 2004).

To manage your weight safely and for the long-term, you should plan meals and snacks throughout the day.

The Major Components of a Successful, Life-long Weight Management Plan Are:

1. Recognizing you have control over what you eat.
2. Recognizing that you can choose to make time to exercise.
3. Ensuring that the calories you consume are equal to the calories you spend if you want to stay the same weight.
4. Ensuring that the calories you consume are less than the calories you spend if you want to lose weight.
5. Ensuring that the calories you consume are more than the calories you spend if you want to gain weight.

HEALTHIER GROCERY SHOPPING

To be a healthier grocery shopper, spend more time in the outer aisles of the store where fresh foods are kept. Spend less time in the middle aisles where packaged foods, snacks, and soft drinks are stocked.

Shopping List

- Fresh vegetables and fruits should make up the largest part of your healthy foods grocery list.
- Purchase grain and cereal products made from whole grains, not from refined flours. This part of your list includes whole grain breads, whole grain pastas, and whole grain breakfast cereals. Whole grains are important for vitamins, minerals, and for fiber, which is often lacking in modern diets. Read labels to look for 100 percent whole grain or 100 percent whole wheat to ensure you are getting whole grain products.
- Your protein and meat choices should consist mostly of fish, poultry, and lean meats. Eggs, nuts, seeds, and legumes are also good sources of protein. Choose fresh and frozen unbreaded meats and fish. Avoid breaded, deep-fried convenience foods that you put in the oven. They are high in fats and sodium.
- Beverages should be kept simple. Water, low-fat milk, juices, and herbal teas are all good choices. If you choose soft drinks, choose diet ones to avoid extra sugar.
- Dairy products should include low fat milk, yogurt, and cheese. If you do not want cows' milk, choose soy and rice beverages, calcium fortified orange juice, or goats' milk and cheese.
- Be careful with dressings, cooking oils, and condiments. They are sneaky sources of refined sugar and poor quality oils. Read labels to choose dressings made with olive oil, canola oil, or walnut oil. Choose low-fat mayonnaise for your sandwiches, and choose canola oil and olive oil for cooking.
- Frozen foods are a convenient way to keep vegetables on hand. Prepared meals that you can pop into the microwave or oven can be convenient and healthy if you choose low-fat versions with good portion sizes. Read labels and chose frozen foods wisely. Avoid frozen pizzas, pocket-sandwiches, deep-fried appetizers, and breaded foods.
- Foods in cans and jars are also very convenient. Look for low-sodium soups, vegetables, and sauces. Avoid high-fat gravies and high-calorie foods like canned spaghetti and ravioli products.
- For sandwiches, choose peanut butter or other nut butters, low-fat turkey slices, or sliced roast beef. Avoid processed lunch meats, sausages, and hot dogs.
- Do not load up on high calorie treats and desserts. Choose fresh fruits, healthy nuts, seeds, and whole grain crackers for snacks.

Reading Food Labels

When you go grocery shopping, take time to read the nutrition labels on your purchases. Compare nutrients and calories in one food to those in another. Pay attention to the serving size and the servings per container. All labels list total calories in a serving size of the product. Compare the total calories in the product that you choose with others like it; choose the one that is lowest in calories.

Product: **Check for:**

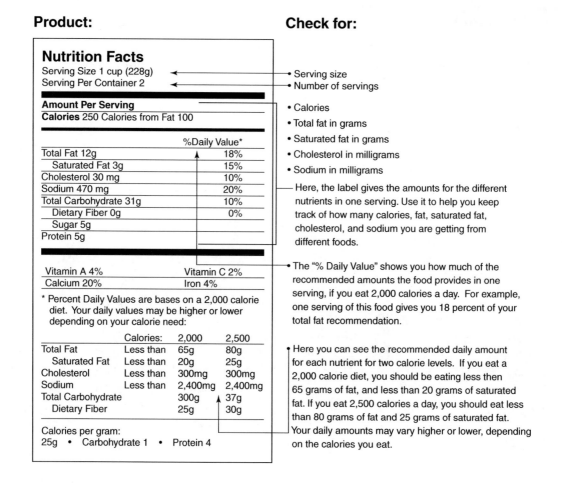

The "Nutrition Facts" label contains this information:

Serving size: If you eat double the serving size listed, you need to double the calories, fat, and nutrients. If you eat half the size shown, cut the calories and nutrients in half.

Calories: This is very helpful to know if you're cutting calories to lose weight.

Total Fat: The label gives you the number of grams of fat per serving (so you can track your daily intake) and the number of calories from fat. If you are overweight or trying to lose weight, you should set a goal of an overall intake of no more than 25 to 35 percent of your total calories from fat, with less than 7 percent as saturated fat and less than 1 percent as trans fat.

Saturated fat: It is a key nutrient for raising your blood cholesterol and your risk of heart disease and stroke. Eat less saturated fat!

Cholesterol: Too much cholesterol in your diet may lead to too much of it in your blood.

Too much cholesterol in your blood can lead to heart disease and stroke. It is best to eat less than 300 mg each day. People with heart disease, high LDL cholesterol levels or who are taking cholesterol medication should consume less than 200 mg of cholesterol per day.

Sodium: Watch for both natural and added sodium. Ordinary table salt is sodium chloride, 40 percent sodium by weight. Healthy adults should take in less than 2,300 mg of sodium each day, which is equal to about 1 teaspoon of salt. African Americans, middle-aged and older adults, and people with high blood pressure need less than 1,500 mg per day.

Total Carbohydrate: Emphasize fruits, vegetables, and whole-grain breads and cereals.

Dietary Fiber: Fruits, vegetables, whole grains, peas, and beans are good sources and can help reduce the risk of heart disease.

Protein: Most animal protein contains fat and cholesterol; therefore, eat small portions.

Vitamins and Minerals: Eating a variety of foods will help you reach your daily goal of 100 percent of vitamin A, vitamin C, calcium, and iron.

Daily Value: The daily values are guides for people who eat 2,000 calories each day. If you eat more or less than that, your daily value may be higher or lower. Choose foods with a low percent daily value of fat, saturated fat, cholesterol, and sodium. Try to reach 100 percent of the daily value of total carbohydrates, dietary fiber, vitamins, and minerals.

EATING HEALTHY ON A BUDGET

Today Americans are paying at the gas pump, but also at the grocery store.

Preparing your own food is one of the best ways to make sure that you are making healthy choices. It is also a great way to save money compared to eating out or buying prepared meals. Eating healthier foods can actually save you money. According to a 2002 study published in the *Journal of the American Dietetic Association,* the researchers found that when families went on weight loss diets, they not only lost weight but also reduced their food budgets. The savings came from reducing portion sizes and from buying fewer of the high-calorie foods that tend to increase the amount spent at the grocery store (Glanz et al., 1998). People tend to spend a lot on those "extras," foods that add calories but little nutritional value, like sodas, bakery items, and chips. The ideal food is nutrient-dense, not calorie-dense, and the least expensive may be fresh, frozen, or canned. Save money by passing on calorie-dense cakes and cookies; instead, opt for seasonal fruit.

Tips for Eating Healthy on a Budget

- Have a light snack before you go grocery shopping, and stick to your grocery list to help avoid impulse purchases or costly mistakes like falling for the displays at the end of the aisles.
- Before you plan your weekly menu, check the ads to see what is on sale and use money-saving coupons.
- Check the food section in your newspaper to find the best buys for the week, based on fresh produce in season. Shop your local farmers' market for great deals on local produce.
- Planning meals around what is on sale can lower your grocery bills, especially if you also use coupons. Stock up on staples when they are on sale.
- Making lunch and taking it with you is a great money-saver and an excellent use of leftovers. Packing your lunch not only saves you money, but also allows you control of all the ingredients so they are healthy and low in calories.
- Using frozen foods may be less expensive than fresh, yet they are equally nutritious. Produce is typically frozen at the peak of ripeness, when nutrients are plentiful. Fish and poultry are often flash-frozen to minimize freezer damage and retain freshness. With frozen foods, you can use only the amount you need, reseal the package, and return it to the freezer.

- Substitute inexpensive, vegetarian sources such as beans, eggs, tofu, and legumes for more expensive meat, fish, or poultry. Eat vegetarian once a week or more to increase your consumption of healthy plant foods while saving money. Eggs are an excellent, inexpensive source of protein that can be eaten for breakfast, lunch, or dinner. Also, think of meat as a "condiment" and use it sparingly. Americans consume far too much animal-based protein, mostly from fatty sources. Eating it as you would a condiment will not only save you money, but help your health.
- Go generic. Consider buying store brands instead of pricier national brands. Read the ingredient list on the label to be sure that you are getting the most for your money.
- Try to concentrate your shopping around the outer aisles of the store and avoid the inner aisles. The outer aisles tend to house the fresh vegetables, meats, eggs, and dairy products. The inner aisles tend to contain mostly processed foods, which are more expensive and less healthy.

HEALTHY EATING OUT

Americans are eating out more than ever. When dining out, it is easy to eat more calories and fat as well as food that is less healthy.

Tips for Healthy Eating Out

- Practice eating small portions. At a typical restaurant, a single serving provides enough for two meals. Take half the entrée home or split the meal with a friend. Order an appetizer as a main course instead.
- Go to places where you can order healthy, low-fat meals.
- According to the Center for Science in the Public Interest, soft drinks are the single biggest source of calories in the American diet. One 32-ounce Big Gulp with non-diet cola packs about 425 calories, so one Big Gulp can quickly gulp up a big portion of your daily calorie intake. Try switching to water with lemon or unsweetened iced tea.
- Request items be made without butter or oil. Ask for your vegetables and main dishes to be served without the sauces. If your food is fried or cooked in oil or butter, ask to have it broiled or steamed. Ask to substitute high fat items like french fries for a baked potato or side salad instead.
- Eat a little less at noon to save for a special dinner later, but do not skip meals which can lead to eating too much.
- Eat something 30 minutes before your meal to help be in better control of your choices. Eat a piece of fruit or have a glass of water with lemon.
- Avoid buffets, and all-you-can-eat specials. You will likely overeat to get your money's worth. If you do choose buffet dining, opt for fresh fruits, salads with low-fat dressings, broiled entrées, and steamed vegetables. Resist the temptation to go for seconds, or wait at least 20 minutes after eating to make sure that you are really still hungry before going back up to the buffet.
- Dishes labeled "deep-fried," "pan-fried," "basted," "batter-dipped," "breaded," "creamy," "crispy," "scalloped," "Alfredo," "au gratin," or "in cream sauce" are usually high in calories, unhealthy fats, or sodium.
- Be aware of calorie- and fat-packed salad dressings, spreads, cheese, and sour cream. For example, ask for a grilled chicken sandwich without the mayonnaise.

- Breaded, batter-dipped, and tempura all are fried food, which is heavy in fat. Look instead for lower fat, grilled, broiled, and flame-cooked. Other good choices include entrées that are steamed, poached, roasted, or baked in their own juices.
- For sauces, stick to wine, or thinned, stock-based sauces. Avoid thick butter sauces, béarnaise, Mornay, or sauces that sound creamy.
- If ordering pizza, ask for extra vegetable toppings and forget the meats and extra cheese.
- Count alcohol calories as part of your eating. Alcohol is very high in calories and can prevent us from making healthy food choices.

What to Order When Eating Out

Fast-Food

Be aware that the average fast-food meal can easily run more than 1,000 calories and contain a full day's worth of sodium. Check the nutritional value of foods by asking the restaurant or checking the restaurant's Web site before you go. Choose the salads, water, or diet sodas or the children's portion if you are craving that food. Also, if you eat fast food for one meal, plan around it to cut the rest of the day's calories, sodium, and sugars and increase fruits and vegetables.

- Watch out for words like jumbo, giant, deluxe, biggie-sized, or super-sized. Larger portions mean extra calories and more fat, cholesterol, sodium, and sugar.
- Avoid eating croissants and biscuits because they have lots of extra fat and very little fiber.
- End a meal with sugar-free, fat-free yogurt. Ices, sorbets, and sherbets have less fat, but still have lots of sugar. Bring a piece of fruit from home for your dessert after eating lunch out.
- Be alert for tricky information. For example, a fat-free muffin is fat-free but much higher in sugar than another muffin. Chinese food may seem okay if you order steamed vegetables, but if you use lots of soy sauce you get too much sodium.
- Choose barbequed or broiled and grilled chicken sandwiches—as well as a regular hamburger or roast beef sandwich—instead of jumbo burgers and fried sandwiches.

EATING OUT: HEALTHY AND UNHEALTHY CHOICES

Burger Chains

Healthy Choices	Unhealthy Choices
Regular, single-patty hamburger without mayonnaise or cheese	Double-patty hamburger with cheese, mayonnaise, special sauce, and bacon
Grilled chicken sandwich	Fried chicken sandwich
Veggie burger	Fried fish sandwich
Garden salad with grilled chicken and low-fat dressing	Salad with toppings such as bacon, cheese, and ranch dressing
Egg on a muffin	Breakfast burrito with steak
Baked potato	French fries
Yogurt parfait	Milk shake
Grilled chicken strips	Chicken "nuggets" or tenders
Limiting cheese, mayonnaise, and special sauces	Adding cheese, extra mayonnaise, and special sauces

Fried Chicken Chains

Healthy Choices	Unhealthy Choices
Skinless chicken breast without breading	Fried chicken (original or extra-crispy)
Honey barbeque chicken sandwich	Teriyaki wings or popcorn chicken
Garden salad	Caesar salad
Mashed potatoes	Chicken and biscuit "bowl"
Limiting gravy and sauces	Adding extra gravy and sauces

Taco Chains

Healthy Choices	Unhealthy Choices
Grilled chicken soft taco	Crispy shell chicken taco
Black beans	Refried beans
Shrimp ensalada	Steak chalupa
Grilled "fresco" style steak burrito	Crunch wraps or gordita-type burritos
Vegetable and bean burrito	Nachos with refried beans
Limiting sour cream, guacamole, or cheese	Adding sour cream, guacamole, or cheese

Subs, Sandwich, and Deli Choices

Healthy Choices	Unhealthy Choices
Six-inch sub	Foot-long sub
Lean meat (roast beef, chicken breast, lean ham) or vegetables	High-fat meat such as ham, tuna salad, bacon, meatballs, or steak
One or two slices of lower-fat cheese (Swiss or mozzarella)	The "normal" amount of higher-fat (Cheddar, American) cheese
Adding low-fat dressing or mustard instead of mayo	Adding mayonnaise and special sauces
Adding extra vegetable toppings	Keeping the sub "as is" with all toppings
Choosing whole-grain bread or taking the top slice off your sub and eating it open-faced	Choosing white bread or "wraps" which are often higher in fat than normal

Casual-fare Restaurant Choices

Healthy Choices	Unhealthy Choices
Side salad with low-fat dressing or a side of steamed vegetables	Salads with fried onions, cheeses, meats, and high-fat dressings
Turkey, roast beef, or grilled chicken sandwich	Mayonnaise-heavy tuna or chicken salad sandwich
Baked or grilled fish	Battered or deep-fried fish
Chicken or turkey wraps without mayonnaise or cheese	Extra-large burgers loaded with cheese and sauces

Asian Food Choices

Healthy Choices	Unhealthy Choices
Egg drop, miso, wonton, or hot and sour soup	Fried egg rolls, spare ribs, tempura
Stir-fried, steamed, roasted, or broiled entrees (shrimp chow mein, chop suey)	Battered or deep-fried dishes (sweet and sour pork, General Tso's chicken)
Steamed or baked tofu	Deep-fried tofu
Sauces such as ponzu, rice-wine vinegar, wasabi, ginger, and low-sodium soy sauce	Coconut milk, sweet and sour sauce, regular soy sauce
Steamed brown rice	Fried rice
Edamame, cucumber salad, stir-fried vegetables	Salads with fried or crispy noodles

Italian and Pizza Restaurant Choices

Healthy Choices	Unhealthy Choices
Thin-crust pizza with half the cheese and extra vegetables	Thick-crust or butter-crust pizza with extra cheese and meat toppings
Plain rolls or breadsticks	Garlic bread
Antipasto with vegetables	Antipasto with meat
Pasta with tomato sauce and vegetables	Pasta with cream or butter-based sauce (Alfredo)
Red sauce (marinara, red clam, or marsala)	Entree with side of pasta
Entree with side of vegetables	Fried ("Frito") dishes
Grilled ("Griglia") dishes	Parmigiana, beef lasagna
	Cheese sauce or filling, pesto, carbonara, sausage dishes

Steakhouse

- Trim the fat from broiled meat and order without sauces or gravy.
- A filet, flank, or London broil steak is the leanest cut.

Salad Bar

- Be careful about potato and pasta salads, bacon bits, marinated vegetables, olives, fruits in heavy syrup, and seeds or nuts.
- One ladle of creamy salad dressing can be about 300 calories.
- Select dark, leafy greens, raw vegetables and fruits, lean ham or turkey, and cottage cheese.
- Use fat-free dressing or low-fat dressing in small amounts.

Pizza

- Vegetable pizzas can have half the calories of the "works" type.
- Ask for extra vegetables to replace the meat on pizza.
- You can request half of the cheese as well.

Mexican

- Chicken fajitas, tortillas, and Spanish rice without sour cream and guacamole are often okay choices.
- Go easy on chips and rich or fried items on the menu such as chili rellanos, nachos, chorizo, chimichangas, flautas, and taco bowl salads.

MENU PLANNING IS THE KEY

When you take the time to plan out menus, you can creatively use leftovers, buy only the food you need, and save time and money. Meal planning also makes you think about foods that will satisfy your needs.

Sample Menus for a 2,000 Calorie Food Pattern

Breakfast	Lunch	Snacks	Dinner
(Choose one below)	*(Choose one below)*	*(Choose one below)*	*(Choose one below)*
Breakfast burrito	Roast beef sandwich	1 cup cantaloupe	Stuffed broiled salmon
1 flour tortilla (7" diameter)	*1 whole grain sandwich bun*		*5 ounce salmon filet*
1 scrambled egg (in 1 tsp soft margarine)	*3 ounces lean roast beef*		*1 ounce bread stuffing mix*
	2 slices tomato		*1 tbsp diced celery*
⅓ cup black beans	*¼ cup shredded romaine lettuce*		*2 tsp canola oil*
2 tbsp salsa	*⅛ cup sauteed mushrooms (in 1 tsp oil)*		*½ cup saffron (white) rice*
1 cup orange juice	*1 ½ ounce part-skim mozzarella cheese*		*1 ounce slivered almonds*
1 cup fat-free milk	*1 tsp yellow mustard*		*½ cup steamed broccoli*
	¾ cup baked potato wedges		*1 tsp soft margarine*
	1 tbsp ketchup		*1 cup fat-free milk*
	1 unsweetened beverage		

Breakfast	Lunch	Snacks	Dinner
(Choose one below)	*(Choose one below)*	*(Choose one below)*	*(Choose one below)*
Hot cereal *½ cup cooked oatmeal* *2 tbsp raisins* *1 tsp soft margarine* *½ cup fat-free milk* 1 cup orange juice	Taco salad *2 ounces tortilla chips* *2 ounces ground turkey, sauteed in 2 tsp sunflower oil* *½ cup black beans* *½ cup iceberg lettuce* *2 slices tomato* *1 ounce low-fat cheddar cheese* *2 tbsp salsa* *½ cup avocado* *1 tsp lime juice* 1 unsweetened beverage	½ ounce dry-roasted almonds ¼ cup pineapple 2 tbsp raisins	Spinach lasagna *1 cup lasagna noodles, cooked (2 oz dry)* *⅔ cup cooked spinach* *½ cup ricotta cheese* *½ cup tomato sauce with tomato bits* *1 ounce part-skim mozzarella cheese* 1 ounce whole wheat dinner roll 1 cup fat-free milk

Breakfast	Lunch	Snacks	Dinner
(Choose one below)	*(Choose one below)*	*(Choose one below)*	*(Choose one below)*
1 whole wheat English muffin *2 tsp soft margarine* *1 tbsp jam or preserves* 1 medium grapefruit 1 hard-cooked egg 1 unsweetened beverage	Tuna fish sandwich *2 slices rye bread* *3 ounces tuna (packed in water, drained)* *2 tsp mayonnaise* *1 tbsp diced celery* *¼ cup shredded romaine lettuce* *2 slices tomato* 1 medium pear	1 cup fat-free milk	Roasted chicken breast *3 ounces boneless, skinless chicken breast* 1 large baked sweet potato *½ cup peas and onions* *1 tsp soft margarine* 1 ounce whole wheat dinner roll *1 tsp soft margarine* 1 cup leafy greens salad *3 tsp sunflower oil and vinegar dressing*

Based on *mypyramid.gov*

Sample Weekly Menu Planner

Breakfast (about 300 calories)	Lunch (about 400 calories)	Dinner (about 500 calories)	Snacks (about 150 calories)	Desserts (about 150 calories)
Choose one below	Choose one below	Choose one below	Choose one below	Choose one below

Breakfast (about 300 calories) — Choose one below

- Quick breakfast pizza
Cooking spray
1 egg plus 2 egg whites
1 whole-grain pita (5 inches), toasted
2 tbsp shredded part-skim mozzarella cheese
½ tsp dried oregano
½ cup grapes
Make it: Spray skillet with cooking spray and scramble eggs. Top toasted pita with egg, cheese, and oregano. Broil for 5 minutes, until cheese is bubbling. Serve with grapes.

- Skillet pesto-potatoes and eggs
Cooking spray
¾ cup finely chopped potatoes
1 tbsp prepared pesto
1 whole egg
½ medium grapefruit
Make it: Spray skillet with cooking spray. Add potatoes and cook until golden, about 12 minutes, turning once. Toss potatoes with pesto and put on plate. Spray skillet with cooking spray again, cook egg, and place on top of potatoes. Serve with grapefruit.

- Breakfast burrito
1 Amy's Breakfast Burrito (bought prepared)
1 small peach
Toast with walnut and pear spread
½ cup low-fat cottage cheese
1 tbsp chopped walnuts
½ medium pear, finely chopped
2 tsp honey
1 slice whole-grain bread, toasted

Lunch (about 400 calories) — Choose one below

- Turkey, mozzarella, and basil wrap
2 small (6-inch) whole-grain tortillas
3 ounces turkey
1 1-ounce slice part-skim mozzarella cheese, cut in half
¼ cup chopped fresh basil
1 medium apple
Make it: Fill tortillas with turkey, cheese, and basil. Serve with apple.

- White-bean gazpacho with whole-grain roll
½ cup canned white beans, rinsed and drained
1 medium tomato, finely chopped
1 cup finely chopped cucumber
1 garlic clove, minced
2 tbsp red-wine vinegar
1 cup low-sodium tomato juice
Dash of salt and pepper
1 medium whole-grain roll
Make it: Mix beans, tomato, cucumber, garlic, vinegar, tomato juice, and salt and pepper. Serve with roll.

- Asian tuna salad
¼ cup low-fat plain yogurt
1 tsp wasabi powder
½ lime, juiced
2 tsp olive oil
1 tsp light soy sauce
3 ounces tuna, packed in water
2 cups napa cabbage, shredded
½ cup shredded carrots
¼ cup sliced almonds
Make it: Whisk together yogurt, wasabi, lime juice, olive oil, and soy sauce. Toss with tuna, cabbage, carrots, and almonds.

Dinner (about 500 calories) — Choose one below

- Cashew and coconut tofu stir-fry with brown rice
1 tsp sesame oil
1 1-inch slice ginger, minced
1 garlic clove, minced
2 ounces firm tofu, cubed
1 cup frozen stir-fry vegetables
⅓ cup light coconut milk
2 tbsp cashews, chopped
½ cup microwavable brown rice
Make it: Heat oil, ginger, and garlic in skillet for 1 minute. Add tofu and saute for 8 minutes, turning once or twice. Add vegetables, coconut milk, and cashews; cover and cook another 8 minutes. Microwave brown rice, then top with tofu and vegetable mixture.

- Parmesan pasta with asparagus and white beans
2 ounces uncooked whole wheat pasta
2 tsp olive oil
2 garlic cloves, minced
1 ½ cups bite-size pieces asparagus (about 10 spears)
¼ cup canned white beans, rinsed and drained
4 tbsp grated Parmesan cheese
Make it: Cook pasta. In a pan, saute oil, garlic, and asparagus for 4 minutes. Add beans and cook for 4 more minutes. Toss pasta with bean mixture and parmesan.

- Spinach-ricotta frittata with tossed green salad
Cooking spray
1 ½ cups baby spinach
2 eggs plus 2 egg whites, whisked together
⅓ cup part-skim ricotta cheese
Dash of salt and pepper

Snacks (about 150 calories) — Choose one below

- Spicy peanut spread on celery
1 tbsp peanut butter
Cayenne pepper to taste
½ lime, juiced
4 medium celery stalks
Make it: Mix peanut butter, cayenne, and lime juice. (To soften peanut butter, microwave it for 30 seconds.) Spread on celery.

- Honey-curry dip with carrots
⅓ cup low-fat plain yogurt
1 tsp honey
½ tsp curry powder
1 cup baby carrots
Make it: Mix yogurt with honey and curry powder. Dip carrots.

- Corn chips and salsa verde
10 corn chips
2 tbsp prepared green salsa

- Yogurt with honey and sunflower seeds
6 ounces low-fat plain yogurt
1 tsp honey
2 tsp sunflower seeds
Make it: Mix all ingredients together.

- Mini ham and honey-mustard sandwiches
1 tbsp honey-mustard salad dressing
1 slice whole-grain bread, cut into 4 squares
1 ounce low-fat ham
Make it: Spread honey-mustard dressing on bread and top with ham. (Makes 2 mini sandwiches.)

- Grapefruit spritzer and soy nuts
4 ounces 100-percent grapefruit juice

Desserts (about 150 calories) — Choose one below

- Sauteed strawberry sundae
1 tsp balsamic vinegar
1 tsp honey
¼ cup sliced strawberries
½ cup light vanilla ice cream
Make it: Saute vinegar, honey, and strawberries for 3 minutes. Top ice cream with warm berries.

- Grilled pineapple with gingersnap-crumb topping
3 canned pineapple rings, packed in juice
3 tbsp crushed gingersnap cookies (about 2 small cookies)
Make it: Grill pineapple for 3 minutes on each side. Top with crushed cookies.

- Peach and blackberry crepe
1 small peach, chopped
¼ cup low-fat cottage cheese
1 premade crepe (found in the produce department)
1 tbsp 100-percent blackberry fruit spread
Make it: Mix together peaches and cottage cheese, then roll into crepe. Microwave fruit spread for 30 seconds and drizzle over crepe.

- Ice cream treat
½ cup Breyers Rocky Road Double Churn Light Ice Cream
Dark-chocolate-covered graham crackers
4 small graham-cracker rectangles
2 tbsp semisweet chocolate chips
Make it: Microwave chocolate chips for 30 seconds, until just melted. Spread graham crackers with chocolate and let sit for 10

Make it: Mix cottage cheese, walnuts, pear, and honey (for smoother texture, puree in blender). Spread on toast.

• Waffle with fresh blueberries and lemon syrup

¾ cup blueberries

2 tsp maple syrup

½ lemon, juiced

1 whole-grain frozen waffle (4-inch), toasted

1 8-ounce glass skim or light soy milk

Make it: Mash blueberries with fork and mix with maple syrup and lemon juice. Top waffle with blueberry mixture. Serve with milk.

• Strawberry, banana, and flax smoothie

½ medium banana

½ cup frozen, unsweetened strawberries

1 ½ cups skim milk or light soy milk

2 tbsp ground flaxseed

Make it: Blend all until smooth.

• Takeout!

From Au Bon Pain:

Medium oatmeal

Small fruit cup

• Feta, hummus, and cucumber sandwich

⅔ cup canned chickpeas, rinsed and drained

½ lemon, juiced

1 garlic clove, minced

2 tbsp feta cheese

2 slices whole-grain bread

6 cucumber slices

Make it: With potato masher, mash chickpeas, lemon, garlic, and feta. Spread on bread and top with cucumber. .

• Bruschetta burger with spinach salad

1 vegetarian burger

2 tbsp premade bruschetta spread

1 whole-grain hamburger bun

2 cups baby spinach

2 tbsp vinaigrette

Make it: Heat burger in microwave. Place on bun and top with bruschetta. Serve with spinach tossed with vinaigrette.

• Takeout!

From Taco Bell:

Fresco Ranchero Chicken Soft Taco

Fresco Grilled Steak Soft Taco

Side of guacamole

2 cups romaine lettuce

2 tbsp pine nuts

2 tbsp low-fat Italian dressing

Make it: Spray skillet with cooking spray and saute spinach for 2 minutes, until wilted. Stir in eggs, ricotta, and salt and pepper. Cook over medium heat without stirring for 4 minutes; . then flip frittata and cook for an additional 2 minutes. Serve with lettuce tossed with pine nuts and dressing.

• Curried quinoa salad with grilled shrimp

3 ounces frozen uncooked shrimp, thawed under running water for 5 minutes

1 tsp olive oil

¾ cup water

½ cup quinoa

¼ tsp curry powder

1 tbsp dried cranberries

1 cup chopped cucumbers

2 scallions, chopped

Make it: Toss shrimp with oil. Grill for 6 to 8 minutes, flipping once. Bring water and quinoa to a boil, cover, and simmer for 15 minutes. Stir in curry, cranberries, cucumbers, and scallions. Top with shrimp.

• Takeout!

From Chili's:

Guiltless Chicken Sandwich Meal (with black beans and steamed seasonal veggies)

From Ruby Tuesday:

Petite Sirloin

Creamy Mashed Cauliflower

Fresh Tomato and Mozzarella Salad

8 ounces sparkling water

¼ cup soy nuts

Make it: Stir together grapefruit juice and sparkling water. Serve with soy nuts.

• Crackers and goat cheese

6 whole-grain crackers

½ ounce goat cheese

minutes, until chocolate has hardened.

• Homemade mango-lime sorbet

½ cup frozen mango pieces

2 limes, juiced

1 tbsp honey

Make it: Puree ingredients in a blender until smooth and thick.

• Takeout!

From Starbucks:

Petite Vanilla Bean Scone

Grande Iced Coffee (unsweetened)

Guilt-Free Treats

• 2 Skinny Cow Vanilla and Caramel Skinny Dippers = 160 calories

• 1 VitaBrownie = 100 calories

• 2 Oatmeal Chocolate Chip Cookies (1 pack South Beach Living) = 100 calories

• ¾ cup Ciao Bella Raspberry Sorbetto = 150 calories

• 3 Firecracker Popsicles = 105 calories

• Weight Watchers English Toffee Crunch bar = 110 calories

• 1 Kraft Handi-Snacks Chocolate Pudding = 100 calories

• 1 Nabisco 100 Calorie Packs Mister Salty Milk Chocolate Covered Pretzels = 100 calories

Name _____ Date _____

NUTRITION ASSIGNMENT #10

1. Plan a weekly healthy meal plan for yourself based on your *caloric needs*. *Include healthier versions of fast-food, listed in this chapter and healthy recipes can be found in Chapter 11.* Also write a shopping list of all the ingredients you will need for the week.

Monday	Tuesday	Wednesday	Thursday	Friday	Saturday	Sunday

RESOURCES

Agricultural Research Magazine, "Nutrition Research: Key To Eating Better." *December 1999.*

American Heart Association: *www.americanheart.org*

Bouchard, C. 1997. Genetics of Human Obesity: Recent Results from Linkage Studies. *The Journal of Nutrition* 127, (9):1887S–1890S.

Bray, G. 2002. Predicting Obesity in Adults from Childhood and Adolescent Weight. *The American Journal of Clinical Nutrition.* 76, (3):497–498.

Byers, T., Nestle, M., McTiernan, A. et al. 2002. American Cancer Society guidelines on nutrition and physical activity for cancer prevention: reducing the risk of cancer with healthy food choices and physical activity. *CA: A Cancer Journal for Clinicians.* 52:92–119.

Calle, E. E., Rodriguez, C., Walker-Thurmond, K., Thun, M. J., 2003. Overweight, obesity and mortality from cancer in a prospectively studied cohort of U.S. adults. *New England Journal of Medicine.* 348(17):1625–1638.

Center for Science in the Public Interest: *https://www.cspinet.org/*

Dansinger, M. L., Gleason, A. J., Griffith, J., Selker, H. P., Schaefer, E. J. 2005. Comparison of the Atkins, Ornish, Weight Watchers, and Zone Diets for Weight Loss and Heart Disease Risk Reduction. *Journal of the American Medical Association.* 293:43–53.

Duke University Diet and Fitness Center: *www.dukedietcenter.org*

Fitness magazine, August 2008.

Glanz, K., Basil, M., Maibach, E., et al. 1998. Why Americans eat what they do: taste, nutrition, cost, convenience, and weight control concerns as influences on food consumption. *Journal of the American Dietetic Association.* 98:1118–26.

International Agency for Research on Cancer: *http://www.iarc.fr/*

Jetter, K. M., Cassady, D. L. 2005. The availability and cost of healthier food alternatives. *American Journal of Preventive Medicine.* 30:38–44.

Mitchell, D. C., Shannon, B. M., McKenzie, J., et al. 2005. Lower fat diets for children did not increase food costs. *Journal of Nutrition Education.* 32:100–3.

National Heart Lung and Blood Institute: *http://www.nhlbi.nih.gov/health/public/heart/obesity/lose_wt/shop_lst.htm.*

Nutrition Analysis Tools and System: *http://nat.crgq.com.*

Portion Distortion slide sets: *http://hp2010.nhlbihin.net/portion/.*

Raynor, H. A., Kilanowski, C. K., Esterlis, I., Epstein, L. H. 2002. A cost-analysis of adopting a healthful diet in a family-based obesity treatment program. *Journal of the American Dietetic Association.* 102:645–50.

Spiegel, K., Tasali, E., Penev, P., Van Cauter, E. 2004. Sleep Curtailment in Healthy Young Men Is Associated with Decreased Leptin Levels, Elevated Ghrelin Levels, and Increased Hunger and Appetite. *Annals of Internal Medicine.* 141:846–850.

Stroke Association: *www.StrokeAssociation.org.*

USDA Nutrient Data Laboratory: *www.nal.usda.gov.*

World Health Organization Technical Report Series 916. 2003. Diet, nutrition and the prevention of chronic diseases: report of a joint FAO/WHO Expert Committee. Geneva: World Health Organization: *http://whqlibdoc.who.int/trs/WHO_TRS_916.pdf.*

World Health Organization. 2000. Obesity: preventing and managing the global epidemic. Geneva: WHO.

chapter 11
Healthy Recipes

Tuna-Stuffed Red Pepper Salad

Ingredients:

- 1 medium sweet red bell pepper
- 1 3-ounce can chunk light tuna in water, drained and flaked
- 1 small green onion, sliced (reserve a few slices for garnish, if desired)
- ¼ cup cooked brown rice
- 1 tbsp chopped celery or water chestnuts
- 2 tsp low-sodium soy sauce
- ½ tsp fresh grated ginger
- 2 tsp rice vinegar
- ½ tsp sesame oil
- Salt, to taste

Directions:

Remove stem from red bell pepper and slice in half, lengthwise. Set aside half for another use. In a small bowl, mix together the tuna, green onion, cooked brown rice, and celery or water chestnuts. Add the remaining ingredients and combine. Spoon tuna mixture into the pepper shell and garnish with reserved green onion slices. Serve slices of the red pepper with the tuna filling.

Nutrition Analysis per Serving:

- Calories 228
- Total Fat 4g
- Sat. Fat 0.5g
- Mono Fat 1g
- Trans Fat 0g
- Poly Fat 1.5g
- Carbs 21g
- Dietary Fiber 4g
- Protein 25g
- Sugars 5.5g
- Sodium 758mg
- Cholesterol 25.5mg

Vegetarian Stuffed Peppers
Ingredients:

4 green bell peppers

4 servings brown rice

1 can kidney or any type of bean (low sodium)

Boca or Morningstar vegetable ground crumbles

Salsa or diced tomatoes

Directions:

Core and clean peppers; place in microwave-safe dish with a little water in the bottom until they get somewhat soft. Make brown rice; add kidney or any type of bean and vegetable ground crumbles. Add any seasoning depending on desired spiciness and some salsa or diced tomatoes. Stuff mixture into peppers and bake for about 45 minutes or until lightly browned on top.

Nutrition Analysis per Serving:

Calories 350

Protein 24g

Carbs 58g

Total Fat 1.5g

Sodium 630mg

Fiber 12g

Chowder
Ingredients:

1 tbsp vegetable oil

1 cup onion, chopped

1 celery stalk, chopped

1 carrot, chopped

⅛ tsp cayenne pepper

½ tsp cumin

1 garlic clove, minced

2 cups fresh corn kernels (approximately 4 ears)

2 large, fresh tomatoes, chopped

1 small zucchini, quartered and sliced

1-½ cup water

1 tsp salt

2 cup fresh spinach, chopped

1-½ cup milk (1%)

2 tbsp fresh cilantro, minced

Directions:

Heat oil in a heavy 2-quart saucepan; sauté onion, celery, carrots, cayenne, cumin, and garlic until tender (5 to 7 minutes). Add corn, tomatoes, zucchini, water, and salt to sautéed vegetables. Bring to a boil; reduce heat to low. Cover and simmer for about 30 minutes until corn is tender. Add spinach, milk, and cilantro. Heat 5 minutes more over low heat. Thin with additional milk if necessary.

Nutrition Analysis per Serving:

Calories 189.81

Protein 7.75g

Carbs 30.98g

Total Fat 5.79g

Saturated Fat 1.29g

Cholesterol 5.63mg

Sodium 713.04mg

Fiber 4.79g

Asian Lettuce Wraps

Ingredients:

½ cup reduced-fat peanut butter

¼ cup honey

2 tbsp Hoisin sauce

2 tbsp water

2 tsp fresh lime juice

⅛ tsp ground red pepper

Cooking spray

1 lb skinless, boneless chicken breast halves

12 romaine lettuce leaves

2 cups julienne-cut carrots

1 cup julienne-cut seeded, peeled cucumbers

1 cup fresh sprouts

Directions:

Combine first six ingredients in a bowl and whisk. Set aside. Coat a large, nonstick skillet with cooking spray and place over medium-high heat. Add chicken; thoroughly cook each side until done, cool, then slice into strips. Divide chicken evenly among lettuce leaves; top with carrot, cucumber, and sprouts. Roll up and serve with sauce.

Makes 6 servings (serving size: 2 wraps and 2 tbsp sauce)

Nutrition Analysis per Serving:

Calories 295.61

Protein 24.21g

Carbs 31.87g

Total Fat 9.28g

Saturated Fat 1.96g

Cholesterol 43.85mg

Sodium 369.13mg

Fiber 3.94g

Sautéed Spanish Chorizo

Ingredients:

6 to 8 oz roasted red pepper

4 oz chorizo

3 oz goat cheese

5 to 6 fresh basil leaves

1 clove fresh garlic, finely diced

2 tbsp white wine

Directions:

Roast peppers over an open flame until well charred, then place in a bowl and cover with plastic wrap. When the peppers are cool enough to handle, peel, seed, and julienne them. Dice chorizo into ¼-inch pieces. Heat about 1 ounce olive oil and begin to sauté the chorizo, draining any excess fat. Add roasted peppers, garlic, and white wine, finish with roughly chopped basil, and place into dish. Sprinkle with goat cheese and garnish with basil on top.

Nutrition Analysis per Serving:

Calories 228.77

Protein 11.49g

Carbs 4.53g

Total Fat 17.2g

Saturated Fat 8.47g

Cholesterol 41.74mg

Sodium 685.14mg

Fiber 0.04g

Turkey Wrap
Ingredients:

2 oz honey turkey
3 thin slices red onion
4 thin apple slices
2 slices cheddar cheese
1 tbsp garlic mayo (1 cup mayonnaise with 1 clove minced garlic)
1 red pepper tortilla

Makes 2 servings

Nutrition Analysis per Serving:

Calories 200
Protein 12g
Carbohydrates 9g
Total Fat 13g
Saturated Fat 4g
Cholesterol 50mg
Sodium 711mg
Fiber 5g

Chocolate Custard Cake .
Ingredients:

Cake:

Vegetable oil spray
14-oz can nonfat sweetened condensed milk
Egg substitute equivalent to 5 eggs
½ cup 1% milk
½ cup Splenda
¼ cup nonfat or low-fat chocolate syrup

Topping:

1-¼ cup seedless all-fruit preserves (fruit of choice)
10 oz fresh or frozen blueberries, thawed
1 tbsp powdered sugar (optional)

Directions:

Preheat the oven to 350° F. Spray an 8-inch nonstick round cake pan with vegetable oil spray. Cut a circle of parchment paper or wax paper to fit the bottom of the pan. Place paper in pan. If using wax paper, spray the top with vegetable oil spray.

In a large bowl, whisk together all cake ingredients. Pour into prepared pan.

Place the pan in the middle of a 12- × 17- × 1-inch jellyroll pan and fill jellyroll pan half full with warm water, or place cake pan in a baking pan (the bottom of a broiler pan works well), and add warm water to a depth of 1 inch.

Bake for 40 to 45 minutes, or until a toothpick inserted in the center of the cake comes out clean. Remove cake pan from water and let cool on a wire rack for 10 minutes. Carefully invert onto a plate (it is not necessary to loosen sides first) and remove paper.

Let cool for 15 minutes. While cake is cooling, heat preserves in a small saucepan over low heat, stirring occasionally.

Top the cake with a thin coating of the preserves. Sprinkle with about half of the blueberries. Cut the cake into 10 pie-shaped slices. Spoon remaining preserves on each dessert plate. Place each cake slice on preserves. Top with remaining blueberries, then dust lightly with powdered sugar.

For a more formal presentation, place blueberries in a ring around the top of the cake before cutting. Sprinkle any remaining berries on the dessert plates.

Makes 12 servings

Nutrition Analysis per Serving:

Calories 269.13

Protein 6.15g

Carbs 60.87g

Total Fat 0.28g

Saturated Fat 0.14g

Cholesterol 3.98mg

Sodium 115.19mg

Fiber 0.82g

Vegetable Stew
Ingredients:

2 tbsp water

1 cup zucchini, thinly sliced

1-¼ cups yellow squash, thinly sliced

½ cup green bell pepper, cut into 2-inch strips

¼ cup celery, cut into 2-inch strips

¼ cup onion, chopped

½ tsp caraway seeds

⅛ tsp garlic powder

1 medium tomato, cut into 8 wedges

Directions:

Add first six ingredients to a heavy, nonstick skillet over medium heat. Cover and cook 4 minutes, or until vegetables are just tender. Add remaining ingredients, reduce heat to low, cover, and cook another 2 minutes.

nutrition Analysis per Serving:

Calories 38
Fat 0.7g
Cholesterol 0mg
Protein 1.6g
Carbohydrates 8.6g
Fiber 2.6g
Sugar 4.6g
Sodium 13mg

Honey Dijon Spinach Salad

Ingredients:

1 lb. spinach leaves, washed and torn into pieces, tough stems discarded

2 cups mushrooms, sliced

1 cup cherry tomatoes, cut in half

¼ cup fat-free honey dijon dressing

Directions:

Combine spinach, mushrooms, and tomatoes in a salad bowl. Pour dressing over salad and toss.

nutrition Analysis per Serving:

Calories 67
Fat 0.7g
Cholesterol 0mg
Protein 4.6g
Carbohydrates 13.4g
Fiber 4.5g
Sugar 5.2g
Sodium 245mg

Baked Beans

Ingredients:

2 bacon slices (or turkey bacon) cut into 1-inch pieces (optional)

1-¼ lbs canned baked beans

⅓ cup onion, chopped

2 tbsp plus 2 tsp brown sugar, firmly packed

2 tsp molasses

1-¼ tsp Worcestershire sauce

¼ tsp dry mustard

Directions:

Heat a heavy, nonstick skillet over medium high heat. Sauté bacon 5 to 7 minutes, stirring frequently until crisp. Drain and discard drippings. Stir in remaining ingredients. Cover, reduce heat to medium low and **simmer** 15 minutes.

Nutrition Analysis per Serving:

Calories 183
Fat 0.7g
Cholesterol 0mg
Protein 7g
Carbohydrates 41.8g
Fiber 7.3g
Sugar 20.3g
Sodium 585mg

Sweet Whipped Potatoes
Ingredients:

¾ lb sweet potatoes, peeled and cut into 1-inch pieces
½ lb baking potatoes, peeled and cut into 1-inch pieces
¼ cup cottage cheese
¼ cup evaporated skim milk
¼ tsp salt (optional), or to taste
⅛ tsp pepper

Directions:

Place potatoes in steamer basket over boiling water. Cover and **steam** about 15 minutes or until tender. Remove potatoes from pan. Transfer to a mixing bowl. While potatoes are cooking, place cottage cheese in a food processor or blender and process until smooth. Transfer cottage cheese and remaining ingredients to potatoes. Beat with an electric mixer at medium speed until mixture is smooth.

Nutrition Analysis per Serving:

Calories 178
Fat 1.0g
Cholesterol 3mg
Protein 5.7g
Carbohydrates 37.2g
Fiber 3.7g
Sugar 8.0g
Sodium 91mg

Potato Salad

Ingredients:

1-¾ lbs small new potatoes

1 large egg, hard-cooked, peeled and chopped

3 tbsp fat-free mayonnaise

3 tbsp nonfat sour cream

¼ cup dill relish

1 tbsp scallions, finely chopped

2 tbsp prepared mustard

1 tsp dried tarragon

Directions:

Place potatoes in a steamer basket over boiling water. Cover pan and **steam** about 20 minutes or until just tender. Drain potatoes and rinse under cold running water to cool. Combine remaining ingredients with salt and pepper to taste in a bowl. Peel potatoes and cut into ½-inch dice cubes and gently toss with egg mixture. Serve potato salad chilled or at room temperature.

This recipe serves 8 people. Due to the nature of this recipe, it adjusts the number of servings in multiples of 8 only.

Nutrition Analysis per Serving:

Calories 123

Fat 1.2g

Cholesterol 36mg

Protein 3.5g

Carbohydrates 25g

Fiber 2.0g

Sugar 4.2g

Sodium 170mg

Chicken Teriyaki

Ingredients:

2 chicken breasts, whole, split in half

½ cup soy sauce

¼ cup dry sherry

1 tbsp sugar

1 clove garlic, chopped

½ tsp ground ginger

Directions:

Arrange chicken, skin side up, in a single layer in a shallow dish. Combine soy sauce, sherry, sugar, garlic, and ginger in a jar with a tight-fitting lid. Shake vigorously and pour over chicken. Marinate in refrigerator 2 hours, turning once or twice. Preheat broiler. Remove chicken from marinade. Spray rack in broiler pan with vegetable spray. Transfer chicken to rack. Broil about 10 minutes about 6 inches from heat, turning once and basting with marinade.

Nutrition Analysis per Serving:

Calories 141

Fat 1.4g

Cholesterol 53mg

Protein 22.9g

Carbohydrates 6.5g

Fiber 0.3g

Sugar 4.6g

Sodium 1889mg

Japanese Soba Noodle Salad
Ingredients:

11 ounces soba noodles

2 scallions, minced

1 tbsp plus 1 tsp fresh parsley, chopped

2 tsp mirin wine

2 tbsp lemon juice

¾ tsp fresh ginger, grated

¾ tsp garlic, pressed

1 tbsp plus 1 tsp yellow or white miso paste

1-¼ tsp sesame seeds

Directions:

Cook soba noodles in a large pan of boiling water about 5 minutes. Drain and rinse with cold water. Combine noodles, scallions, and parsley in a bowl. Combine next 4 ingredients in a separate bowl. Then mix in miso, working out the lumps with the back of a spoon. Thin if necessary with a little water, drop by drop. Combine with noodle mixture and chill. Garnish with sesame seeds.

Nutrition Analysis per Serving:

Calories 110

Fat 1.1g

Cholesterol 0mg

Protein 5.4

Carbohydrates 21.0g

Fiber 2.0g

Sugar 1.3g

Sodium 259mg

Orange-Grilled Chicken with Herbs

Ingredients:

2 cloves garlic, crushed

¾ tsp orange peel, grated

¼ tsp fresh thyme, minced

¼ tsp fresh rosemary, minced

Freshly ground black pepper

1 lb boneless chicken breast fillets, skin attached

⅓ cup fresh orange juice

1 tbsp plus 1 tsp vinegar

2 tsp Worcestershire sauce

Directions:

Combine the first 5 ingredients in a small bowl to make the herb mixture. Take each chicken breast and slip your fingers between the skin and flesh of the chicken, leaving the skin attached. Slide some of the herb mixture under the skin of each breast, pulling the skin back over each breast when finished. Prepare an outside grill with an oiled rack set 4 inches above the heat source.

On a grill, set the heat to high. Mix together the orange juice, vinegar, and Worcestershire sauce in a small bowl. Grill the chicken breasts for 3–4 minutes on each side, turning once and basting with the orange juice mixture, until the chicken is cooked through. Remove the skin before eating.

Nutrition Analysis per Serving:

Calories 140

Fat 1.5g

Cholesterol 66mg

Protein 26.5g

Carbohydrates 3.6g

Fiber 0.1g

Sugar 2.4g

Sodium 102mg

Pasta Salad

Ingredients:

2 cups cooked corkscrew macaroni

1-⅓ cups chopped tomatoes

⅔ cup canned sweet corn kernels

⅔ cup canned black beans or red kidney beans, drained and rinsed

⅓ cup red onions, or purple onions

3-½ tbsp chopped red bell pepper

3-½ tbsp chopped green bell pepper

3-½ tbsp chopped yellow bell pepper

1-¼ tsp vinegar

¾ tsp lemon juice

¾ tsp olive oil

¾ tsp Italian herb seasoning

1 tbsp plus 1 tsp grated Parmesan or Romano cheese

⅛ tsp orange zest, optional

⅛ tsp salt (optional)

⅛ tsp black pepper (optional)

Directions:

Mix all ingredients in a large bowl. Keep refrigerated until served (up to 24 hours).

Nutrition Analysis per Serving:

Calories 173

Fat 2.3g

Cholesterol 1mg

Protein 7.2g

Carbohydrates 32.5g

Fiber 5.5g

Sugar 6.3g

Sodium 132mg

Shrimp Salad

Ingredients:

    1 lb cooked shrimp, thawed and drained

    1 cucumber, peeled, seeded and thinly sliced

    12 radishes, thinly sliced

    4 scallions, sliced

    ½ cup white wine vinegar

    1 tbsp sugar

Directions:

Combine all ingredients in a bowl and toss well. Chill.

Nutrition Analysis per Serving:

    Calories 181

    Fat 2.6g

    Cholesterol 196mg

    Protein 27.7g

    Carbohydrates 11.4g

    Fiber 2.1g

    Sugar 8.0g

    Sodium 200mg

Grilled Pork Tenderloin

Ingredients:

    4 pork tenderloin chops

    ½ tsp coarsely ground black pepper

    ⅔ cup orange marmalade

    ¼ cup fresh mint, chopped

    ¼ cup lite soy sauce

    4 cloves garlic, crushed

Directions:

Prepare grill or turn on broiler. Butterfly tenderloin by cutting a lengthwise slit two-thirds of the way into each tenderloin, without cutting all the way through. Place tenderloin between 2 sheets of plastic wrap. Flatten slightly with a mallet or other heavy flat object. Sprinkle with pepper. Combine remaining ingredients in a small nonreactive saucepan. Brush mixture over tenderloin. Set aside remaining marmalade mixture. Grill or broil tenderloin about 8 minutes per side, basting frequently with marmalade mixture. Heat remaining marmalade mixture over medium heat about 1 minute, stirring until warm. Serve tenderloin with marmalade mixture.

Nutrition Analysis per Serving:

Calories 220

Fat 2.3g

Cholesterol 35mg

Protein 13.9g

Carbohydrates 38.3g

Fiber 0.4g

Sugar 34.9g

Sodium 589mg

Lower Fat Biscuits

Ingredients:

1-⅓ cups reduced fat buttermilk baking mix

½ cup skim milk

Directions:

Preheat oven to 450° F. Combine both ingredients in a bowl and stir until a soft dough forms. If dough is too sticky, gradually stir in enough baking mix (up to 1 tbsp plus 1 tsp) to make dough easy to handle. For rolled biscuits: Turn dough onto surface dusted with baking mix. Roll in baking mix to coat. Knead 10 times. Roll to ½-inch thick. Cut with a 2-½ inch cutter. Place on an ungreased cookie sheet. For drop biscuits: Do not knead dough. Drop by spoonfuls onto an ungreased cookie sheet. Bake 7 to 9 minutes or until golden brown.

Nutrition Analysis per Serving:

Calories 162

Fat 2.6g

Cholesterol 1mg

Protein 4.1g

Carbohydrates 29.8

Fiber 0.5g

Sugar 3.5g

Sodium 480mg

Sweet and Sour Chicken

Ingredients:

3 tbsp cornstarch

1-2/3 cups canned Asian or chicken stock

¼ cup vinegar

¼ cup sugar

1 lb boneless skinless chicken breast halves, cut into cubes

1 small green or red bell pepper, cut into 2-inch strips

1 medium carrots, sliced

½ lb unsweetened pineapple chunks, drained

4 cups hot cooked rice

Directions:

Combine first 4 ingredients in a bowl until smooth. Set aside. Heat a heavy nonstick skillet over medium high heat. Stir-fry chicken 5 to 8 minutes, in batches if necessary, or until browned. Set chicken aside.

Stir cornstarch mixture and add to skillet. Cook until mixture boils and thickens, stirring constantly. Return chicken to pan. Add pepper, carrot, and pineapple. Reduce heat to low. Cover and cook 5 minutes or until chicken is no longer pink. Serve over rice.

This recipe serves 4 people. Due to the nature of this recipe, it adjusts the number of servings in multiples of 4 only.

Nutrition Analysis per Serving:

Calories 494

Fat 2.8g

Cholesterol 66mg

Protein 33.8g

Carbohydrates 81.2g

Fiber 2.2g

Sugar 21.4g

Sodium 412mg

Grilled Chicken Kabobs
Ingredients:

¼ cup water

2 tbsp soy sauce

2 tbsp lemon juice

1 tbsp honey

¼ tsp garlic powder

¼ tsp ground ginger

4 boneless skinless chicken breast halves, cut into 1-½ inch pieces

1 green bell pepper, seeded and cut into 1-½ inch pieces

1 onion, quartered

8 large cherry tomatoes

Directions:

Combine first 6 ingredients in a glass baking dish. Add chicken and turn to coat. Cover and marinate at least 2 hours in refrigerator. Prepare grill. Remove chicken from marinade and boil marinade 10 minutes in a saucepan. Alternate chicken and vegetables on skewers. Grill 6 inches from medium-hot coals 15 to 20 minutes, or until done, turning and basting often with marinade.

Nutrition Analysis per Serving:

Calories 323

Fat 3.7g

Cholesterol 106mg

Protein 46.4g

Carbohydrates 28.2g

Fiber 5.0g

Sugar 18.1g

Sodium 611mg

Broccoli with Bread Crumbs
Ingredients:

1 lb broccoli florets

2 tsp unsalted butter

½ cup seasoned bread crumbs

2 tbsp parsley, finely chopped

Directions:

Place broccoli in a steamer basket over boiling water. Cover saucepan and steam 5 to 6 minutes or until bright green and tender.

Drain and transfer to a serving dish. Keep warm. Melt butter in a heavy nonstick skillet over medium heat. Add bread crumbs and stir until butter is absorbed. Sprinkle broccoli with bread crumbs and parsley. Toss lightly.

nutrition Analysis per Serving:

Calories 104

Fat 2.7g

Cholesterol 5mg

Protein 5.6g

Carbohydrates 16.4g

Fiber 4.0g

Sugar 2.5g

Sodium 428mg

Chicken Marsala
Ingredients:

1-¼ tsp olive oil

¾ medium onion, chopped

1 lb boneless skinless chicken breast halves, pounded to ¼-inch thickness

⅔ cup dry Marsala wine

½ cup chicken stock, low-fat, low-sodium

2 tsp cornstarch, or arrowroot powder

salt and pepper

Directions:

In a large skillet over medium-high heat, heat the oil. Add the onion and sauté for 5 minutes. Add the chicken and cook on each side for 5 minutes. Add the wine and cook for about 4 minutes until the wine looks syrupy. In a small cup, dissolve the cornstarch or arrowroot powder in the stock. Add to the chicken and cook until the sauce is thickened, about 2 minutes. Add salt and pepper to taste.

nutrition Analysis per Serving:

Calories 187

Fat 3.0g

Cholesterol 66mg

Protein 27.3g

Carbohydrates 4.8g

Fiber 0.4g

Sugar 2.3g

Sodium 175mg

Corn Muffins

Ingredients:

1 egg, lightly beaten

1 cup low-fat milk

½ tsp vanilla extract

2 tbsp vegetable oil

½ cup cornmeal

¾ cup flour

¼ cup sugar

1-½ tsp baking powder

½ tsp salt (optional)

Directions:

Preheat oven to 400° F. Combine egg, milk, vanilla, oil, and cornmeal in a mixing bowl. Mix thoroughly. Let stand 10 minutes. Sift remaining ingredients together in another bowl. Add to cornmeal mixture. Mix thoroughly, without overworking. Fill greased muffin tins ⅔ full with batter. Bake 15 minutes, or until tester comes out clean when inserted in center of muffin. Cool 3 minutes in pan before turning muffins out. This recipe serves 12 people.

Nutrition Analysis per Serving:

Calories 96

Fat 3.1g

Cholesterol 16mg

Protein 2.3g

Carbohydrates 14.9g

Fiber 0.6g

Sugar 5.3g

Sodium 17mg

Low-Fat Coffee Cake

Ingredients:

⅓ cup brown sugar, packed

½ tsp ground cinnamon

1-¾ cups reduced-fat buttermilk baking mix

¾ cup skim milk

¼ cup sugar

1 tbsp unsalted butter, melted

1 egg

Directions:

Preheat oven to 375° F. Prepare streusel topping by combining first 2 ingredients in a bowl until crumbly. Set aside. Combine remaining ingredients in another bowl and stir until blended. Spread in a greased 9-inch round pan. Sprinkle with streusel topping. Bake 18 to 23 minutes or until golden brown.

Nutrition Analysis per Serving:

Calories 150
Fat 3.0g
Cholesterol 22mg
Protein 2.8g
Carbohydrates 28.0g
Fiber 0.3g
Sugar 14.2g
Sodium 262mg

Bean Soup
Ingredients:

1 tbsp Extra Virgin Olive Oil
1 medium onion, coarsely chopped
1 medium carrot, peeled and diced
1 celery stalk, trimmed, diced
3 cloves garlic, chopped finely
3 cups vegetable broth
¼ cup ground flaxseed
15-ounce can cooked beans (Navy or Great Northern), washed and drained
Salt and pepper, to taste
Fresh chopped parsley, for garnish

Directions:

Preheat your stockpot, then add oil, onion, carrot, and celery. Over medium heat, sauté these vegetables for 5 to 8 minutes, until the pieces are lightly browned. Add the garlic, and continue to sauté for another minute.

Add the ground flaxseed and the vegetable broth, then simmer the whole mixture covered for about 15 minutes, being careful to keep the pot from reaching a boil. Add beans, salt, and pepper (to taste), and continue cooking for about 5 minutes more. Ladle into serving bowls and garnish with fresh parsley. Accompany each bowl with a slice of whole grain bread for a satisfyingly filling meal.

Nutrition Analysis per Serving:

Calories 176

Fiber 8g

Carbohydrates 23g

Calcium 85mg

Protein 9g

Sodium 589mg

Fat 6g

Cholesterol: 0g

Veggie Quiche
Ingredients:

2 whole eggs

6 egg whites

¾ cup skim milk

1 oz low-fat cheddar cheese, shredded

1-½ cup raw spinach

¾ cup raw, chopped green pepper

¾ cup raw, chopped onion

¾ cup raw, chopped zucchini squash

¾ cup tomato, diced

1 tbsp minced garlic

Dash of salt and pepper

Directions:

Preheat oven to 375° F. Cook spinach according to directions. Drain. Spray 9-inch pie pan with cooking spray to prevent sticking. Combine eggs and milk with a wire whisk in a large mixing bowl. Mix in the green pepper, onion, squash, tomatoes, garlic, salt, and pepper. Fold in the shredded cheddar cheese. Pour all ingredients into 9-inch pie pan. Bake at 375° F for 25 to 30 minutes until knife comes out clean.

Nutrition Analysis per Serving:

Calories 83

Protein 10g

Carbs 6g

Total Fat 2g

Saturated Fat 1g

Cholesterol 76mg

Sodium 167mg

Fiber 1g

Pumpkin Muffins

Ingredients:

½ cup ground flaxseed

2 tsp baking soda

1 tsp cloves

1 tsp cinnamon

½ tsp salt

1 cup chopped nuts

Optional: ½ cup semi-sweet chocolate chips

Directions:

Preheat oven to 350° F and mix the dry ingredients together.

2 cups pumpkin

½ cup plain yogurt

¾ cup honey

1 tsp molasses

2 eggs

Beat the eggs and mix together with other wet ingredients. Mix the wet and dry ingredients together. Place in greased muffin tins. Bake for 20 to 25 minutes until dry to an inserted toothpick. Makes approximately 15 muffins.

Nutrition Analysis per Serving:

Calories 240

Carbohydrates 34g

Protein 6g

Dietary fiber 5g

Total fat 11g

Spanish Omelet

Ingredients:

5 small potatoes, peeled and sliced

1 tbsp olive oil or vegetable cooking spray

½ medium onion, minced

1 small zucchini, sliced

1-½ cup green/red peppers, sliced thin

5 medium mushrooms, sliced

3 whole eggs, beaten

5 egg whites, beaten

Pepper and garlic salt with herbs, to taste

3 ounces shredded part-skim mozzarella cheese

1 tbsp parmesan cheese

Directions:

Preheat oven to 375° F.

Cook potatoes in boiling water until tender. In a nonstick pan, add oil or vegetable spray and warm at medium heat. Add the onion and sauté until brown. Add vegetables and sauté until tender but not brown. In a medium mixing bowl, slightly beat the eggs and egg whites, pepper, garlic salt, and mozzarella cheese. Stir egg-cheese mixture into the cooked vegetables. Oil or spray a 10-inch pie pan or ovenproof skillet. Transfer potatoes and eggs mixture to pan. Spread with parmesan cheese and bake omelet until firm and brown on top, about 20–30 minutes.

Nutrition Analysis per Serving:

Calories 242

Carbohydrates 18g

Protein 19g

Fat 9g

Beef or Turkey Stew

Ingredients:

1 lb lean beef or turkey breast cut into cubes

Whole wheat flour

¼ tsp salt (optional)

¼ tsp pepper

¼ tsp cumin

1-½ tbsp olive oil

2 cloves of garlic, minced

2 medium onions, sliced

2 stalks celery, sliced

1 medium red/green bell pepper, sliced

1 medium tomato, finely minced

5 cups of beef or turkey broth, fat removed

5 small potatoes, peeled and cubed

12 small carrots

1-¼ cups green peas

Directions:

Preheat oven to 375° F.

Mix the whole wheat flour with salt, pepper, and cumin, and roll the beef or turkey cubes in the mixture. Shake off excess flour. In a large skillet, heat the olive oil over medium-high heat. Add the beef or turkey cubes and sauté until nicely brown, about 7–10 minutes. Place the beef or turkey in an ovenproof casserole. Add minced garlic, onions, celery, and peppers to the skillet and cook until vegetables are tender, about 5 minutes.

Stir in the tomato and broth. Bring to a boil and pour over the turkey or beef pieces. Cover the casserole tightly and bake for 1 hour at 375° F. Remove from the oven and stir in the potatoes, carrots, and peas. Bake for another 20–25 minutes, or until tender.

Nutrition Analysis per Serving:

Calories 326

Carbohydrates 21g

Protein 27g

Fat 15g

Caribbean Red Snapper
Ingredients:

2 tbsp olive oil

1 medium onion, chopped

½ cup chopped red pepper

½ cup carrots, cut in strips

1 clove garlic, minced

½ cup dry white wine

¾ lb red snapper fillet

1 large tomato, chopped

2 tbsp pitted ripe olives, chopped

2 tbsp crumbled feta cheese or low-fat ricotta cheese

Directions:

In a large skillet, heat olive oil over medium heat. Add onion, red pepper, carrot, and garlic; sauté 10 minutes. Add wine and bring to boil. Push vegetables to one side of the pan. Arrange fillets in a single layer in center of skillet. Cover; cook for 5 minutes. Add tomato and olives. Top with cheese. Cover; cook 3 minutes, or until fish is firm but moist. Transfer fish to serving platter; garnish with vegetables and pan juices.

Nutrition Analysis per Serving:

Calories 193
Carbohydrates 3g
Protein 22g
Fat 11g

Two Cheese Pizza
Ingredients:

Whole wheat flour
1 can (10 oz) refrigerated pizza crust
2 tbsp olive oil
½ cup low-fat ricotta cheese
½ tsp dried basil
1 small onion, minced
2 cloves garlic, minced
¼ tsp salt (optional)
4 ounces shredded part-skim mozzarella cheese
2 cups chopped mushrooms
1 large red pepper, cut into strips

Directions:

Preheat oven to 425° F.
Spread whole wheat flour over working surface. Roll out dough with rolling pin to desired crust thickness. Coat cookie sheet with cooking spray. Transfer pizza crust to cookie sheet. Brush olive oil over crust. Mix the ricotta cheese with the dried basil, onion, garlic, and salt; spread this mixture over crust. Sprinkle crust with mozzarella cheese. Top cheese with mushrooms and red pepper. Bake at 425° F for 13 to 15 minutes until cheese melts and crust is deep golden brown. Cut into 8 slices.

Nutrition Analysis per Serving:

Calories 351
Carbohydrates 34g
Protein 18g
Fat 16g

Eggplant Lasagna

Ingredients:

1 medium onion, sliced

1 clove garlic, minced

1 large tomato, sliced very thin

1 cup canned crushed tomatoes

1-½ tsp dried basil

1-½ tsp dried oregano

¼ tsp salt (optional)

1 medium eggplant, sliced very thin

8 ounces shredded part-skim mozzarella cheese

Directions:

Preheat oven to 425° F.

In a medium nonstick skillet, heat olive oil over medium heat. Sauté onion until tender, about 2–3 minutes. Transfer to an 8×8 or 9×13 baking dish. Sauté the garlic for 1 minute. Add the crushed tomato, basil, oregano, and salt, and cook gently over medium-low heat for 10 minutes. Spread a layer of this mixture over the onion layer. Add a layer of eggplant and follow with a layer of tomato. Sprinkle ⅓ of the mozzarella cheese over top. Repeat layers of eggplant, tomato, and cheese until you use all ingredients. Finish with a layer of mozzarella cheese. Cover with aluminum foil and bake for 25 minutes, or until vegetables are tender. Uncover and bake 10 to 15 minutes, or until layer of cheese is light brown.

Nutrition Analysis per Serving:

Calories 219

Carbohydrates 5g

Protein 16g

Fat 15g

Rice with Chicken, Spanish Style

Ingredients:

2 tbsp olive oil

2 medium onions, chopped

4 garlic cloves, minced

2 stalks celery, diced

2 medium red/green peppers, cut into strips

1 cup chopped mushrooms

2 cups uncooked rice

1 3-lb chicken, cut into 8 pieces, skin removed

1 tsp salt (optional)

3-½ cups chicken broth, fat removed

4 cups water Saffron or Sazón, for color

3 medium tomatoes, chopped

1 cup frozen peas

1 cup frozen corn

1 cup frozen green beans

Olives or capers for garnish, if desired

Directions:

Heat the oil over medium heat in a nonstick pot. Add the onion, garlic, celery, green pepper, and mushrooms. Cook over medium heat, stirring often, for about 3 minutes or until tender. Add the rice and sauté for 2 to 3 minutes, stirring constantly until it begins to brown. Add the chicken, salt, chicken broth, water, saffron (Sazón), and tomatoes. Bring the water to a boil, then reduce heat to medium-low and let simmer. Cover the pot and let the casserole simmer until the water is absorbed and rice is tender, about 20 minutes. Stir in the peas, corn, and beans, and cook for 8 to 10 minutes. When everything is hot the casserole is ready to serve. Garnish with olives or capers, if desired.

Nutrition Analysis per Serving:

Calories 330

Carbohydrates 24g

Protein 27g

Fat 14g

Seafood Stew
Ingredients:

6 cups water

10 oz white wine

3 celery stalks, chopped

3 medium carrots, chopped

1 lb large shrimp, washed

1 lb crayfish

2 tbsp olive oil

2 medium onions, chopped

1 medium red pepper, chopped

1 medium green bell pepper, chopped

4 medium tomatoes, chopped

2 tbsp tomato paste

2 tsp chopped fresh thyme

2 tsp chopped fresh oregano

1 lb sea bass, cut into chunks

1 lb small squid, cleaned and sliced

Salt and pepper to taste

Directions:

In a large, non-aluminum saucepan, stir together the water, white wine, celery, and carrots. Bring to a simmer and cook for 5 minutes. Add the shrimp and crayfish and simmer for 3 to 4 minutes. Strain the shellfish and vegetables from the broth and set the broth aside. Peel the crayfish and shrimp and discard the shells. Warm the olive oil in the large saucepan over medium-high heat. Cook the onions and peppers until tender, about 6 minutes. Stir in the tomatoes, tomato paste, thyme, and oregano. Add the reserved broth and bring to a simmer. Stir in the sea bass and squid and simmer for 2 minutes. Return the crayfish, shrimp, and vegetables to the broth and simmer for 1 more minute. Season to taste, ladle into bowls, and serve immediately.

Nutrition Analysis per Serving:

Calories 222

Carbohydrates 3g

Protein 36g

Fat 8g

RESOURCES

American Diabetes Association's. 1996. *Flavorful Seasons Cookbook: Great-Tasting Recipes for Winter, Spring, Summer and Fall.* McGraw-Hill Companies.

Golden Valley Flax: *www.flaxhealth.com.*

National Institutes of Health: *www.ndep.nih.gov.*

Today's Diet and Nutrition: *www.todaysdiet&nutrition.com.*

INDEX

A

AAP. *See* American Academy of Pediatrics
Acceptable macronutrient distribution ranges
    (AMDR), 40
Acesulfame-K, 112
Added sugars, 37
Aerobic exercise, 136
Agatston, Arthur, 104
Agricultural practices, 117
Alcohol, cancer patient and, 70
Alpha-linolenic acid (ALA), 58
Alzheimer's disease, 4
American Academy of Pediatrics (AAP), 80
American Dietetic Association (ADA), 40, 87
American Heart Association, 44, 60
    dietary recommendations, 61–62
American Psychologist, 152
Amino acids, 44
Angina, 56
Anorexia, 85
Antioxidants, 47, 60–61, 70
    beta-carotene, 60
    lutein, 60
    lycopene, 61
    selenium, 61
    Vitamin A, 61
    Vitamin C, 61
    Vitamin E, 61
Apple body shape, 132–133
Artificial sweeteners, 112
Asian lettuce wraps, 183–184
Aspartame, 112
Atkins diet, 35, 36, 101–102
Atkins, Robert, 101
Autoimmune disease, 64

B

Baked beans, 187–188
Bananas, 100
Basal metabolic rate, 7
Beans, 42
Bean soup, 199–200
Beef or turkey stew, 202–203
BHA preservative, 109
Binge eating, 86
Bio-electrical impedance analysis (BIA), 136
Bisphenol A (BPA), 116
Blood glucose level, 65, 66
Blood serum cholesterol, 43
Body composition, 136–137
Body fat percentage, 135–137
Body image, 86–87
Body mass index (BMI), 133–134
Body temperature, 7
Bone density, 67. *See also* Osteoporosis
Bottled water, 113–114
    environmental impact of, 116
Bran, 38
Bratman, Steven, 86
Breast feeding, 7, 79
Broccoli with bread crumbs, 196–197
Budget, healthy eating and, 167–168
Bulimia, 85–86
Bureau of Labor Statistics, 9

C

Calcium, 48
    osteoporosis and, 68
    toddlers and, 80–81
Caliciviris, 125

Calories
    defined, 5
    formula for determining daily requirements, 8
    kilocalories, 5
Campylobacter, 125
Cancer, 4, 36, 59
    alcohol and, 70
    diet and, 69–71
    fat and, 70
    fiber and, 70
    fruits and vegetables and, 70
    nitrates and, 70
Cancer-causing ingredients, 109–110
Carbohydrates, 18, 26, 35–40
    complex, 38–39
    fiber and, 40–41
    misconceptions, 147–148
    simple, 37–38
    types of, 37–38
    whole grains and, 38–39
Cardiovascular disease (CVD), 58. *See also* Heart
    disease
Caribbean red snapper, 203–204
Cayenne pepper, 100
Celiac disease, 73–74
    symptoms of, 73
Centers for Disease Control and Prevention
    (CDC), 64, 79, 121
Chemotherapy
    diet and, 71
    side effects of, 71
Chicken marsala, 197
Chicken teriyaki, 189–190
Child/adolescent nutrition, 82
Chloride, 49
Chocolate custard cake, 185–186
Cholesterol, 42–43
    heart disease and, 57
Chowder, 182–183
Chronic pain, 59
Cinnamon, 100
Citrus fruits, 100
Clinical dietician, responsibilities of, 11
Clinton, Bill, 46
Complex carbohydrates, 38–41
Corn muffins, 198
Coronary artery disease (CAD), 4, 56
    fiber and, 60
Culture, food selection and, 10

D

Dairy products, 25, 28
DASH (Dietary Approaches to Stop
    Hypertension) diet, 63
Davis, Adelle, 2
Death, leading causes of in United States, 3
Department of Health and Human Services
    (HHS), 20
Depression, 59
Diabetes, 4, 59, 64–69
    diabetes food pyramid, 66–67
    diagnosing, 64
    gestational, 65
    misconceptions, 145–146
    Type I, 64–65
    Type II, 64, 65
Diabetes food pyramid, 66
Diastolic pressure, 62
Dietetics, 12
Diet
    cancer patient and, 69–71
    diabetes and, 64–67, 64–69
    diseases and, 55
    gluten intolerance, 72–73
    heart disease and, 56–62
    HIV/AIDS and, 72
    hypertension and, 62–63
Dietary cholesterol, 43
Dietary fiber, 60
Dietary guidelines. *See also* USDA food guidance,
    history of USDA's, 17
Dietary Guidelines for Americans, 20
Dietary Reference Intake (DRI), 40, 63
Dietary Supplement Health and Education
    Act, 46
Diets. *See* Eating plans
Diet strategies, 163–164
Diet trends, 95–104
Disaccharides, 37, 38
Discretionary calories, 22–28
Disease, poor diet and, 4
Disease prevention, nutrition and, 3–4
Diverticular disease, 40–41
DNA, 69, 95
Docosahexaenoic acid (DHA), 58

E

Eat, Drink and be Healthy: The Harvard Medical School Guide to Healthy Eating, 18
Eating disorders, 84–86
    amenorrhea and, 85
    anorexia, 85
    binge eating, 86
    bulimia, 85–86
    female athlete triad syndrome and, 84–85
    orthorexia nervosa, 86
    osteoporosis and, 85
    signs and symptoms of, 85
    treatment for, 86
Eating out, 168–172
    healthy vs. unhealthy choices, 169–172
    tips for healthy, 168–169
Eating plans, 101–104
    Atkins diet, 101–102
    calories comparison in, 160–162
    Slim-Fast diet, 102
    South Beach diet, 104
    Weight Watchers, 102–103
    Zone diet, 103–104
E. coli, 117, 125
Eggplant lasagna, 205
Eicosapentaenoic acid (EPA), 58
Electrolytes, 49
Endosperm, 38
Energy
    content of in food, 5–6
    nutrition and, 2
Energy in/energy out, 22
Enriched grain, 39
Environmental Protection Agency (EPA), 114, 118
Exercise, 58, 90, 139

F

Farmer's market, 97, 98
Fast food, 160, 169
Fat hormones, 138–139
Fat, misconceptions, 146–147
Fat-burning foods, 100
Fats, 18, 25–26, 41–44. *See also* Lipids
    cancer patient and, 70
Fat-soluble vitamins, 47
FD&C Citrus Red No. 2, 109
Female athlete triad syndrome, 84–85
    signs and symptoms of, 85

Fetal alcohol spectrum disorders (FASD), 88
Fiber, 38, 40–41
    cancer patient and, 70
    diverticular disease and, 40–41
    insoluble, 40
    soluble, 40
Fluoride, 49
Folate, 48
Folic acid, 39
    pregnancy and, 87
Food
    convenience and, 9
    cost factor in selection of, 9
    culture and, 109
    as emotional comfort, 9–10
    energy in, 5–6
    interactions with medicines, 73–74
    selection, 8–11
    serving size, 23
Food additives, 109
Food and Drug Administration (FDA), 44, 95, 99, 115, 117, 118
Foodborne illness, 121–125
    Centers for Disease Control (CDC) estimates, 121
    food temperature and, 123
    most common diseases, 125
    risk factors, 121, 123
    riskiest foods, 123
    steps for avoiding contamination, 124
Food for Young Children, 17
Food Guide Pyramid, 17, 18, 20
    for kids, 27–28
Food labels, 40, 41, 44, 99
    organic, 120–121
    reading, 165–167
Food supply dangers, 109–125
    acesulfame-K, 112
    additives, 109
    aspartame, 112
    cancer-causing ingredients, 109–110
    drinking water, 113–115
    foodborne illness, 121–125
    food coloring, 113
    high fructose corn syrup, 111–112
    meat and fish, 117–118
    Monosodium Glutamate (MSG), 110–111
    olestra, 112
    plastics and, 116–117
    sodium nitrate, 112
    trans fat, 113

Frolich, Theodor, 2
Fructose, 37
Fruits, 24, 28
    cancer patient and, 70
Functional food, 99–100
    examples of, 99
    health claims and, 99

G

Galactose, 37
Garlic, 100
Genetically modified organisms (GMO), 95
Genetically modified organisms (G.M.O.),
    consequences of, 95
Germ, 38
Gestational diabetes, 65
Ghrelin, 139
Ginger, 100
Glucose, 37, 64, 65
Gluten intolerance, 73–74
Government food programs, 20
Grilled chicken kabobs, 196
Grilled pork tenderloin, 193–194

H

Harvard Heart Letter, 153
Harvard's Healthy Eating Pyramid, 18
Healthy eating
    benefits of, 159
    budget and, 167–168
    eating out and, 168–172
    grocery shopping for, 165–167
    menu planning, 172–175
    mindful eating and, 162–163
    strategies, 163–164
    symptoms of lack of, 159–160
Healthy Eating Pyramid, 19
    tips for using, 19–20
Heart attack, 56
    symptoms of, 56
Heart disease, 4, 55, 56–62
    fiber and, 60
    heart attack symptoms, 56
    reducing risk of, 56–57
    saturated fats and, 57
    types of, 56
Heart failure, 56

Height, 7
Height and weight charts, 132
High blood pressure. *See* Hypertension
High density lipoprotein (HDL), 43, 57
High fructose corn syrup (HFCS), 111–112,
    148–150
    health dangers of, 112
High-quality proteins, 44
HIV/AIDS, 72
    diet and, 72
    exercise and, 72
    weight and, 72
Holst, Axel, 2
Honey Dijon spinach salad, 187
Hunt, Caroline, 17
Hypertension, 4, 55, 60, 62–63
    DASH diet, 63
    dietary recommendations for, 62–63
    measuring, 62
Hypothalamus, 50

I

Infant nutrition, 79–80
Influenza, 4
Ingredients to avoid, 109-113. *See also* Food supply
    dangers
Insoluble fiber, 40, 60
Insulin, 65, 138, 146
International Agency for Research on Cancer
    (IARC), 109
International Journal of Obesity, 100
Iodine, 49
Iron, 39, 49
    toddlers and, 81

J

Japanese soba noodle salad, 190–191
Journal of the American Medical Association, 60, 90
Jungle, The, 117

K

Ketones, 36
Ketosis, 36
Kidney failure, 36
Kidney stones, 36
Kilocalories, 5

L

Lactation, 7
Lactose, 38
Leptin, 138–139
Linoleic fatty acid (omega-6), 42
Linolenic fatty acid (omega-3), 42
Lipids, 41–44
    cholesterol, 42–43
    saturated fats, 41–42
    unsaturated fats, 42
Lipoprotein, 43
Low density lipoprotein (LDL), 43, 57, 59
Lower fat biscuits, 194
Low-fat coffee cake, 198–199
Low-quality proteins, 44
Lutein, 60
Lycopene, 61

M

Malnutrition, 3
Maltose, 38
McCollum, E. V., 2
Meat Inspection Act of 1906, 117
Medication interactions with food, 73–74
Mellanby, Edward, 2
Menu planning, 172–175
    sample menus, 172–173
    sample weekly planner, 174–175
Mercury, 118
Mindful eating, 162–163
Minerals, 48
    major, 48–49
    nutrition and, 3
    trace, 49
Monosaccharides, 37
Monosodium Glutamate (MSG), 110–111
Monounsaturated fats, 25, 42
MSG symptom complex, 110–111
Muscle, nutrition and, 2
My Plate, 30
MyPyramid, 21–22
Myths, nutrition, 145–154

N

Nalgene water bottles, 117
National Institutes of Health (NIH), 3
National Nutrition Conference, 17

Natural Resources Defense Council, 114
Natural sugars, 37
Nephritis, 4
New England Journal of Medicine, 36
Niacin, 39
Nitrates, cancer patient and, 70
Nutrients, 4–8, 35–50
    carbohydrates, 5, 35–40
    defined, 4
    energy-yielding, 5
    essential, 5
    lipids, 5
    minerals, 5
    protein, 5
    vitamins, 5
    water, 5
Nutrition
    benefits of proper, 1–3
    cancer patient and, 69–71
    child/adolescent, 82
    defined, 2
    disease prevention and, 3–4
    healthy diet characteristics, 10–11
    history of, 2
    importance of good, 2
    infant, 79–80
    muscle and, 2
    myths, 145–154
    older adults and, 89–90
    pregnancy and, 87–89
    teen, 82–85
    toddler, 80–81
    trends in, 95–104
    vitamins and, 3
Nutrition Labeling and Education Act, 17

O

Obesity, 4, 82, 131–139
    body fat percentage, 136–137
    causes of, 135–137, 137–139
    diseases and, 139
    factors in, 131–132
    measuring, 132–136
    vs. overweight, 134–135
Older adults, nutrition and, 89–90
Olean, 112
Olestra, 112
Omega-3 fatty acid, 42, 58
Omega-6 fatty acid, 42, 59

Orange grilled chicken with herbs, 191
Organic food, 95–98
    benefits of, 96–97
    labeling, 96
    production of, 96
    sustainable agriculture and, 97
Orthorexia nervosa, 86
Osteoporosis, 4, 36, 67–69
    calcium and, 68, 69
    dietary recommendations for, 68
    risk factors, 67–68
    as triad syndrome factor, 85

P

Pain, 59
Parkinson's disease, 59
Pasta salad, 192
Pattern for Daily Food Choices, 17
Pear body shape, 132–133
Phthalates, 116
Physical activity, 7, 8, 23
    moderate, 23
    vigorous, 23
Phytochemicals, 3
Plastic, health dangers of, 116–117
Pneumonia, 4
Polyunsaturated fats, 25, 42
Potassium, 49, 63
Potato salad, 189
Pregnancy, 7, 87–89
    Fetal alcohol spectrum disorders (FASD)
        and, 88
    folic acid and, 87
    nutrition and, 87–88
    pregorexia and, 89
Pregorexia, 89
Processed meats, 110
Protein, 19
Proteins, 23–24, 44–46
    benefits of, 45
Pumpkin muffins, 201
PVC, 116

R

Radiation therapy
    diet and, 71
    side effects of, 71

Recipes, 181–207
    Asian lettuce wraps, 183–184
    baked beans, 187–188
    bean soup, 199–200
    beef or turkey stew, 202–203
    broccoli with bread crumbs, 196–197
    Caribbean red snapper, 203–204
    chicken marsala, 197
    chicken teriyaki, 189–190
    chocolate custard cake, 185–186
    chowder, 182
    corn muffins, 198
    eggplant lasagna, 205
    grilled chicken kabobs, 196
    grilled pork tenderloin, 193–194
    honey Dijon spinach salad, 187
    Japanese soba noodle salad, 190–191
    lower fat biscuits, 194
    low-fat coffee cake, 198–199
    orange grilled chicken with herbs, 191
    pasta salad, 192
    potato salad, 189
    pumpkin muffins, 201
    rice with chicken, Spanish style, 206
    sautéed Spanish chorizo, 184
    seafood stew, 207
    shrimp salad, 193
    Spanish omelet, 202
    sweet and sour chicken, 195
    sweet whipped potatoes, 188
    tuna-stuffed red pepper salad, 181
    turkey wraps, 185
    two cheese pizza, 204
    vegetable stew, 186–187
    vegetarian stuffed peppers, 182
    veggie quiche, 200
Recommended Dietary Allowances (RDAs), 17
    carbohydrates, 40
    lipids, 44
    protein, 45
Refined grains, 39
    reasons for refining, 39
Registered dietician, 11
Rehnborg, Carl, 46
Riboflavin, 39
Roosevelt, Franklin, 17

S

Salmonella, 117, 125
Saturated fats, 25, 41–42, 147
  heart disease and, 57
Sautéed Spanish chorizo, 184
Seafood stew, 207
Sears, Barry, 103
Selenium, 61
Self-esteem, body image and, 86–87
Septicemia, 4
Shrimp salad, 193
Simple carbohydrates, 37–38
  added sugars, 37
  natural sugars, 37
Sinclair, Upton, 117
Skinfold calipers, 136
Skinny fat person, 135-136
Slaughterhouses, 118
Sleep, 164
Stevia, 112
Slim-Fast diet plan, 102
Sodium, 27, 49
Sodium nitrate, 112
South Beach diet, 104
Soy, 60
Soybeans, 100
Spanish omelet, 202
Starch, 38
Stress, 57
  teens and, 82
Stroke, 4
Styrofoam, 117
Sucrose, 38
Sustainable agriculture, 97
Sweet and sour chicken, 195
Sweet whipped potatoes, 188
Systolic pressure, 62

T

Taste, 9
Teen nutrition, 82–85
  eating disorders and, 84–86
  female athlete triad syndrome, 84
  guidelines, 83
Temperature, body, 7

Thermic effect of food, 7
Thiamin, 39
Thin outside, fat inside (TOFI), 135, 151
Toddler nutrition, 80–81
  calcium and, 80–81
  guidelines, 81
  iron and, 81
Total cholesterol level, 57
Toxins, 97
Trace minerals, 49
Trans fats, 26, 43–44, 113, 147
Triglyceride, 56, 57, 58
Tuna-stuffed pepper salad, 181
Turkey wraps, 185
Two cheese pizza, 204
Type I diabetes, 64–65, 145
  symptoms of, 65
Type II diabetes, 4, 65, 146-147
  symptoms of, 65

U

United Nations Children's Fund (UNICEF), 3
Unsaturated fats, 42, 146
USDA food guidance, 17–30
  2010 guidelines, 28–29
  for Americans, 20–21
  discretionary calories, 22–28
  faults of USDA pyramid, 18–20
  history of, 17–18
  My Plate, 30
  MyPyramid, 21–22
U.S. Department of Agriculture (USDA), 17, 20, 37, 95, 117
USDA Organic Seal, 120

V

Vegans, 45
Vegetables, 25, 28
  cancer patient and, 70
Vegetable stew, 186–187
Vegetarian stuffed peppers, 182
Veggie quiche, 200
Vinyl, 116
Vitamin A, 47, 61

Vitamin B12, 48
Vitamin C, 48, 61
Vitamin D, 47, 61
    disease prevention and, 59
Vitamin E, 47, 61
Vitamin K, 47
Vitamins, 46–48
    fat soluble, 46
    history of, 46
    nutrition and, 3
    water soluble, 46

W

Waist circumference, 132–133
Waist-to-hip ratio (WHR), 133
Water, 5, 49–50
    functions of in body, 49
Water safety, 113–115
    bottled vs. tap, 113–114
    guidelines for, 115
Water-soluble vitamins, 48
Weight-bearing exercise, 68, 137

Weight management, 22, 131–139. *See also*
    Obesity
    body fat percentage, 135–137
    body mass index (BMI), 133–134
    components of successful plan, 164
    height and weight charts, 132
    physical activity and, 139
    waist circumference, 132–133
    Weight Watchers, 102–103
    Core plan, 103
    Flex plan, 103
Whole grains, 26–27, 38–39
    labeling, 40
Willet, W., 18

Y

Yale University School of Medicine, 59
Yoga, 137

Z

Zone diet, 103–104